E

In
yo

MW01691896

Emergency Contact:

Police:

Fire:

Doctor:

Poison Control (or 800-222-1222):

Hospital:

PERSONAL INFORMATION

Address:

Telephone:

Cell phone:

Prescribed Medications:

Allergy Information:

Refer to *www.redcross.org/contactcard* for information on the American Red Cross Emergency Contact Card.

American Red Cross' Advisory Council on First Aid and Safety (ACFAS)

In late 1998, the American Red Cross formed an independent panel of nationally recognized health and safety experts known as the Advisory Council on First Aid and Safety, or ACFAS. Drawing on a body of collective expertise from such diverse fields as emergency medicine, occupational health, sports medicine, school health, emergency medical services (EMS) response and disaster mobilization, ACFAS helps establish the standard in first aid care. ACFAS advises the American Red Cross in areas related to the development and dissemination of audience-appropriate information and training in first aid and safety.

A Brief History of First Aid

Clara Barton became familiar with first aid as she worked closely with the International Red Cross to bring the Red Cross to America in 1881. In 1903, as the American Red Cross president, Clara Barton formed a committee to establish first aid instruction among the nation's industrial workers, where conditions were dangerous and accidents and deaths frequent. Her vision was that people would pay a fee for first aid classes and some of the proceeds would help support other Red Cross programs.

Today, the American Red Cross continues that rich tradition by training millions of people each year to save lives and prepare for all types of emergencies.

Table of Contents

Levels of Emergencies iv
Emergency Action Steps v
How to Call 9-1-1 or the Local Emergency Number vii
Life-Threatening Emergencies viii

First Aid Conditions A through Z

Allergic Reaction 1
Bites and Stings 2
Breathing Emergencies 6
Bruises 9
Burns 10

Choking 15
Cuts, Scrapes and Bleeding 25
Diabetic Emergency 27
Drowning 28
Embedded Object 30
Fainting 31
Frostbite and Hypothermia 32

Head, Neck and Back Injuries 35
Heart Attack/Cardiac Arrest/CPR/AED 37
Heat-Related Emergencies 51
Muscle, Bone and Joint Injuries 53
Poisoning 56
Seizures 58
Shock 59
Stroke 60
Tooth (Knocked Out) 62

Emergency Preparedness

Earthquakes 63
Fires, Residential 65
Floods 67
Hurricanes 69
Thunderstorms 71
Tornadoes 73
Preparing for Emergencies 75
First Aid Kit Contents 80

Levels of Emergencies

Life-threatening emergencies

are the most time-critical emergencies. In these situations, always call 9-1-1 or the local emergency number as quickly as possible and begin care.

Urgent emergencies

are sudden, serious conditions that should be monitored closely because they can quickly become life threatening. Quite often, a call to 9-1-1 or the local emergency number is required.

Everyday emergencies

are minor emergencies that need your attention, but are less urgent. These situations rarely require you to call 9-1-1 or the local emergency number.

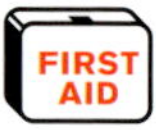

This icon appears throughout this guide and denotes suggested items found in a First Aid Kit.

EMERGENCY ACTION STEPS

Follow the three Emergency Action Steps when responding to an emergency.

1. **CHECK:** CHECK the scene and the person.
2. **CALL:** CALL 9-1-1 or the local emergency number.
3. **CARE:** CARE for the person.

WHEN AND HOW TO CALL 9-1-1

If you are alone, you may have to decide whether to first CALL 9-1-1 or give care before you call. Sometimes a conscious person will tell you not to CALL 9-1-1. You may not always be sure what to do.

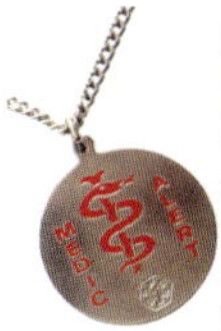

If the person is unconscious, stay calm and CALL 9-1-1 or the local emergency number immediately. Look for a medical identification bracelet or necklace.

IF YOU ARE ALONE

Call First

If you are alone, *Call First*, that is, CALL 9-1-1 or the local emergency number before giving care, for—

- An unconscious adult or adolescent (12 years or older).
- A child or infant who you see collapse suddenly.
- An unconscious infant or child known to be at high risk for heart problems.

Call First situations are likely to be **cardiac emergencies,** such as sudden cardiac arrest, except in children who collapse suddenly.

Care First

If you are alone, *Care First,* that is, give 2 minutes of care, then call 9-1-1 or the local emergency number for—

- An unconscious person younger than 12 years old.
- Any victim of drowning.

Care First situations are likely to be related to **breathing emergencies**.

If you are alone and have to leave the person for any reason—

- Such as to call for help or get an automated external defibrillator (AED), place the person in a recovery position. This will help the airway remain open and clear if the person vomits.

Recovery Position

If the person is unconscious but breathing normally (irregular, gasping or shallow breaths are not effective breaths) and a head, neck or back injury is not suspected—

- Place the person in a recovery position.

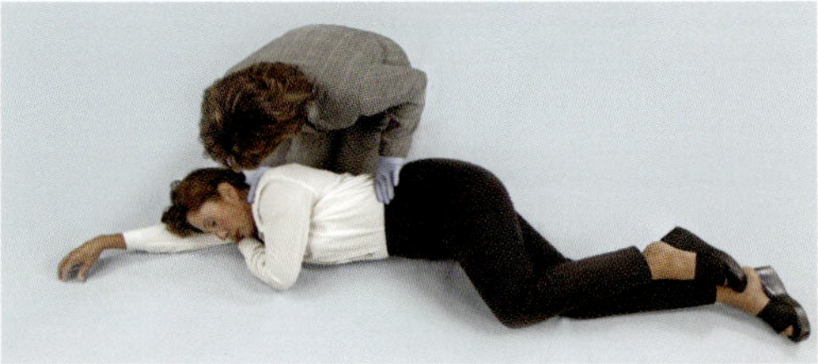

If a head, neck or back injury is suspected—

- Move the person to his or her side while keeping the head, neck or back in a straight line by placing the person in a modified High Arm In Endangered Spine (H.A.IN.E.S.) position.

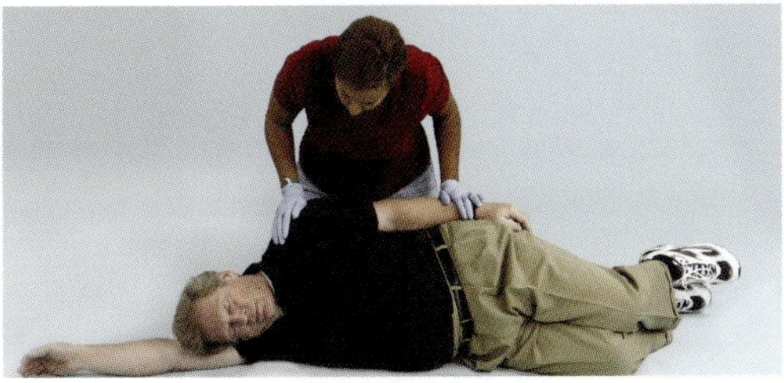

HOW TO CALL 9-1-1 OR THE LOCAL EMERGENCY NUMBER

Stay calm and provide the following information when calling 9-1-1:

- Your name
- The phone number from which you are calling
- What happened
- Your exact location (including intersections, landmarks, building name and/or apartment number)
- How many people are injured
- The condition of the injured people
- What help (first aid) is being given

After you have given all the information to the dispatcher, do not hang up until the dispatcher tells you to.

LIFE-THREATENING EMERGENCIES

These are the most time-critical emergencies. Always CALL 9-1-1 or the local emergency number as quickly as possible and begin care if the person—

- Is or becomes unconscious.
- Has trouble breathing or is breathing in a strange way (see BREATHING EMERGENCIES, page 6).
- Has chest discomfort, pain or pressure that lasts more than 3 to 5 minutes, or goes away and comes back (see HEART ATTACK/ CARDIAC ARREST/CPR/AED, page 37).
- Is bleeding severely (see CUTS, SCRAPES AND BLEEDING, page 25).
- Has a severe burn (see THERMAL BURNS, page 11).
- Has pressure or pain in the abdomen that does not go away.
- Is vomiting blood or passing blood.
- Has seizures, a severe headache or slurred speech.
- Appears to have been poisoned (see POISONING, page 56).
- Has injuries to the head, neck or back (see HEAD, NECK AND BACK INJURIES, page 35).
- Has possible broken bones (see MUSCLE, BONE AND JOINT INJURIES, page 53).
- Is a victim of electric shock (see ELECTRICAL BURNS, page 12).

Also call immediately for any of these situations:

- Fire or explosion
- Downed electrical wires
- Swiftly moving or rapidly rising water
- Presence of poisonous gas
- Vehicle collisions
- People who cannot be moved easily

FIRST AID CONDITIONS A TO B

FIRST AID A-B

ALLERGIC REACTION

What to look for:

- Trouble breathing
- Feeling of tightness in the chest and throat
- Swelling of the face, neck and tongue
- Rash or hives
- Dizziness or confusion

What to do:

- CHECK the scene to make sure it is safe.
- CHECK the person carefully for swelling and breathing problems.
- If you suspect that a person is showing signals of poisoning, call the National Poison Control Center at 800-222-1222. If the person is unconscious or having trouble breathing or if another life-threatening emergency is present, CALL 9-1-1 or the local emergency number. (For other Life-Threatening Emergencies, see page viii.)

Note: For a *severe* allergic reaction, if the person has a prescribed epinephrine auto-injector, you may assist with administration if you are trained to do so and local and state protocols allow.

INSECT BITES/STINGS

What to look for:

- Stinger may be present
- Pain
- Swelling
- Possible allergic reactions (Go to ALLERGIC REACTION, page 1)

What to do:

- Remove stinger:
  - If bee sting, remove it by scraping away with a flat surface like a credit card.
  - Otherwise, try to remove with tweezers. FIRST AID
- Wash wound.
- Cover with dressing.
- Apply ice or a cold pack. FIRST AID
- Watch for signals of severe allergic reaction. (Go to ALLERGIC REACTION, page 1.)

SPIDER BITES/SCORPION STINGS

What to look for:

- Bite mark
- Swelling
- Pain
- Nausea and vomiting
- Trouble breathing or swallowing. (Go to ALLERGIC REACTION, page 1.)

What to do:

- Wash wound.
- Cover with gauze.
- Apply ice or a cold pack. FIRST AID
- CALL 9-1-1 or the local emergency number.

MARINE-LIFE STINGS

What to look for:

- Possible marks
- Pain
- Swelling
- Possible allergic reaction. (Go to ALLERGIC REACTION, page 1.)

What to do:

- If jellyfish—soak area in vinegar.
- If stingray—soak area in hot water (not scalding) until pain goes away.
- Clean and bandage wound.
- CALL 9-1-1 or the local emergency number, if necessary. (Go to LIFE-THREATENING EMERGENCIES, page viii.)

SNAKE BITES

What to look for:

- Bite mark
- Pain
- Swelling

What to do:

If bitten by Pit Viper (rattlesnake, copperhead, cottonmouth)—

- CALL 9-1-1 or the local emergency number.
- Wash wound.
- Keep bitten part still and lower than the heart.

If bitten by Elapid Snake (Coral Snakes)—

- Follow above care steps and—
  - Apply elastic roller bandage to fit snug but not tight.
  - Check feeling, warmth and color of limb before and after applying bandage.
  - Begin wrapping at the point farthest from the heart.

ANIMAL BITES

What to look for:

- Bite mark
- Pain
- Bleeding

What to do:

- If bleeding is minor—wash wound.
- Control bleeding.
- Apply triple antibiotic ointment or cream if no known allergies or sensitivities. FIRST AID
- Cover with dressing.
- Get medical attention if wound bleeds severely or if you suspect the animal has rabies.
- CALL 9-1-1 or the local emergency number or contact animal control personnel.

Rabid animals may drool, appear partially paralyzed or act aggressively or in a strange way.

TICK BITES AND LYME DISEASE

What to look for:

- Rash starts as a small red area at the site of the bite; may appear a few days or a few weeks after the bite
- Fair skin: the center may be lighter in color and the outer edges red and raised (bull's-eye appearance)
- Dark skin: the area may look black and blue
- Fever, headache, weakness
- Flu-like joint and muscle pain

What to do:

- Wear disposable gloves, then grasp tick with tweezers (fine-tipped, pointed, nonetched, nonrasped) close to skin and pull slowly.
- DO NOT try to burn tick off.
- DO NOT apply petroleum jelly or nail polish to tick.
- If you cannot remove tick, or if its mouth-parts remain embedded, get medical care.
- Wash bite area with soap and water.
- Apply antiseptic or triple antibiotic ointment if available or cream (if no known allergies or sensitivities).
- If rash or flu-like signals appear, see your health-care provider immediately.

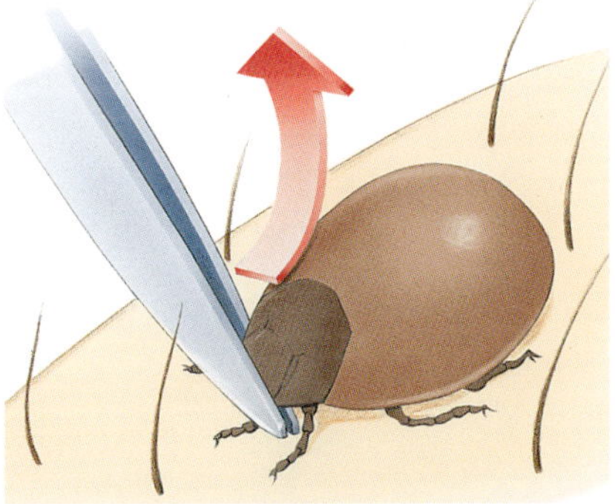

BREATHING EMERGENCIES

The American Red Cross strongly recommends that you take a course in cardiopulmonary resuscitation (CPR) to learn what to do for a breathing emergency.

What to look for:

- Trouble breathing
- Shortness of breath
- Skin appears pale or bluish
- Dizziness or lightheadedness
- Pain in the chest or tingling in hands, feet or lips
- Unusually moist or cool skin

What to do:

- CHECK the scene and the person.
- Send someone to CALL 9-1-1 or the local emergency number.

If person is conscious—

- Have the person rest in a comfortable position.
- Check and care for other conditions you find. (Go to TABLE OF CONTENTS, page iii.)

If person is unconscious—

- Tilt head back and lift chin to open the airway.
- Look, listen and feel for signs of life (movement and breathing) for no more than 10 seconds.

If no breathing, give 2 rescue breaths.

If breathing, place in recovery position and monitor signs of life. (Go to RECOVERY POSITION, page vi.)

If no breathing and no other signs of life—

Adult—

- Begin CPR or use an AED if one is immediately available and you are trained to do so. (Go to CPR—ADULT, page 39, or AED—ADULT, page 41.)

Child—

- Begin CPR or use an AED if one is immediately available and you are trained to do so. (Go to CPR—CHILD, page 44, or AED—CHILD, page 46.)

Infant—

- Begin CPR if you are trained to do so. (Go to CPR—INFANT, page 49.)

Use a CPR breathing barrier FIRST AID if one is available.

STOMA

A stoma is a surgically made breathing hole in the neck.

What to do:

- CHECK for breathing at the stoma.
- When giving rescue breaths, breathe into the stoma in the same way you would give breaths at the mouth. You may have to cover the person's mouth and nose if you do not see the chest rise or if you hear air escape when you breathe into the stoma.

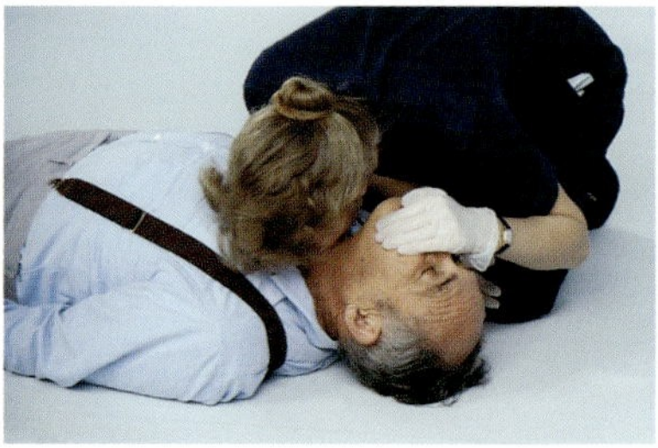

BRUISES

What to do:

- Get permission to give care.
- Apply ice or a cold pack to help control pain and swelling.

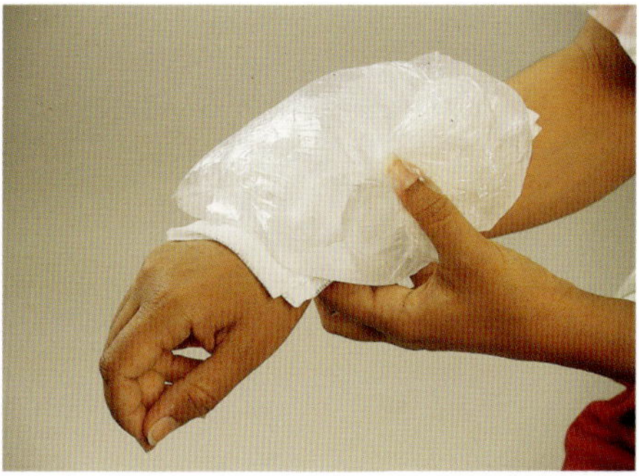

  - Fill a plastic bag with ice or wrap ice with a damp cloth and apply it to the injured area for periods of about 20 minutes.
- Place a cloth, or a thin barrier such as a gauze FIRST AID pad, between the source of cold and skin to prevent injury.
- Elevate the injured part to reduce swelling. DO NOT elevate if it causes more pain.

BURNS

CALL 9-1-1 OR THE LOCAL EMERGENCY NUMBER FOR—

- Burns involving trouble breathing.
- Burns covering more than one body part or large surface area.
- Burns to the head, neck, hands, feet or genitals.
- Burns (other than a very minor one) to a person younger than age 5 or older than age 60.
- Burns resulting from chemicals, explosions or electricity.
- Burns to the mouth and nose.

What to look for:

- Red and dry skin
- Area may swell and is usually painful

How to recognize a deep burn:

- The skin is red and has blisters that may open and weep clear fluid
- May appear brown or black
- Can range from very painful to almost painless

HEAT (THERMAL) BURNS

What to do:

- CHECK the scene and the person.
- Get permission to give care.
- Stop the burning. Remove the person from the source of the burn. Put out flames or remove from source.
- Cool the burn. Use large amounts of cold water.

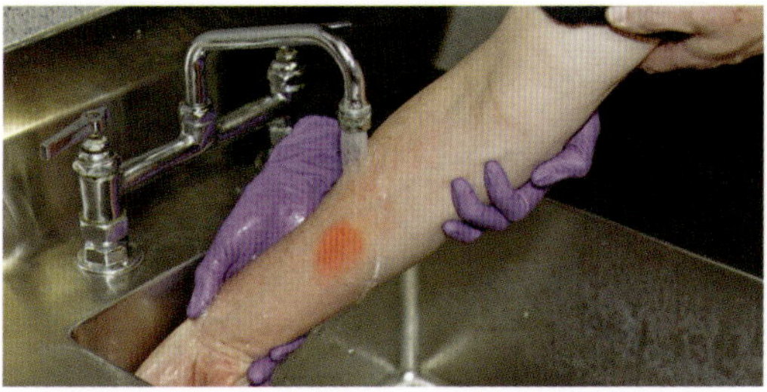

- Cover the burn loosely with a sterile dressing and care for shock. (Go to SHOCK, page 59.)

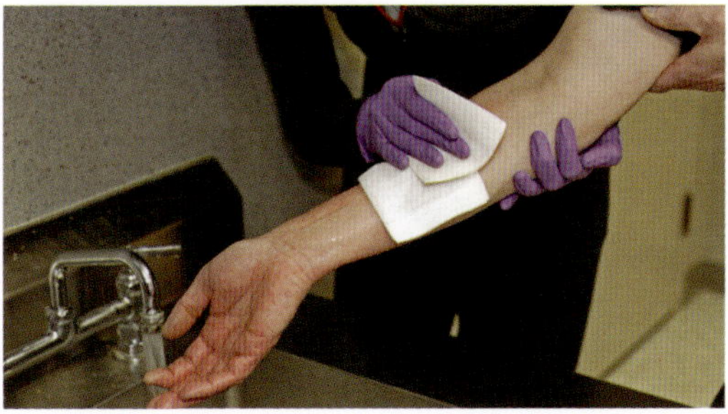

- For a serious burn, call or have someone else CALL 9-1-1 or the local emergency number.

ELECTRICAL BURNS

What to do:

- CHECK the scene and the person.
- Send someone to CALL 9-1-1 or the local emergency number.
- Get permission to give care, if necessary.
- DO NOT go near the person until the power is turned off. If a power line is down, wait for the fire department or power company.
- Be prepared to give CPR or use an AED. (Go to HEART ATTACK/CARDIAC ARREST/CPR/AED, page 37.)
- CARE for shock and thermal burns.

CHEMICAL BURNS

What to do:

- CHECK the scene and the person.
- Send someone to CALL 9-1-1 or the local emergency number.
- Get permission to give care.

For a **dry** chemical—

- Brush dry chemicals off the skin with a gloved hand before flushing with large amounts of cool water.
- Take care not to get any in your eyes or the eyes of the person.
- Remove jewelry and contaminated clothing that may trap chemicals against the skin or on which chemicals may have spilled.

For a **wet** chemical—

- Flush affected areas with large amounts of cool running water for at least 20 minutes or until EMS personnel arrive.
- Always flush away from the body.

SUNBURN

What to look for:

- Red, painful skin with possible blisters
- Possible swelling

What to do:

- CHECK the scene and the person.
- Get permission to give care.
- Cool the burn.
- Protect from further damage by staying out of the sun or wearing sunscreen.
- Protect unbroken blisters with loose bandages FIRST AID and keep broken blisters clean to prevent infection.

FIRST AID CONDITIONS C TO G

FIRST AID C-G

CHOKING

The Red Cross strongly recommends that you take a course to learn how to respond to choking.

CONSCIOUS CHOKING— ADULT AND CHILD

What to look for:

- Clutching throat with one or both hands
- Unable to cough, speak or breathe
- Coughing weakly or making high-pitched sounds

What to do:

- CHECK the scene and the person.
- Send someone to CALL 9-1-1 or the local emergency number and get permission to give care.

If coughing, encourage the person to continue coughing.

If an adult or child is unable to cough, speak or breathe (choking)—

- Lean the person forward and give 5 back blows with the heel of your hand.

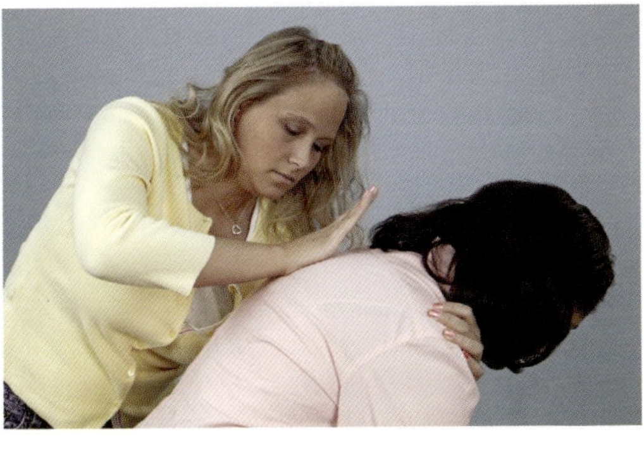

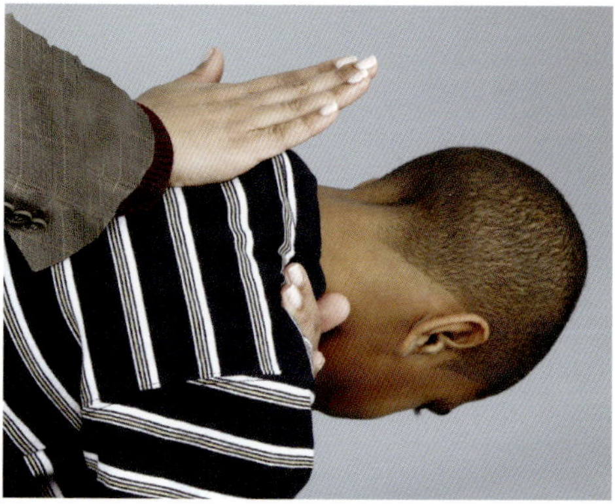

- Give 5 quick, upward abdominal thrusts.
  - Place thumbside of fist against middle of abdomen just above the navel.
  - Grab fist with the other hand.

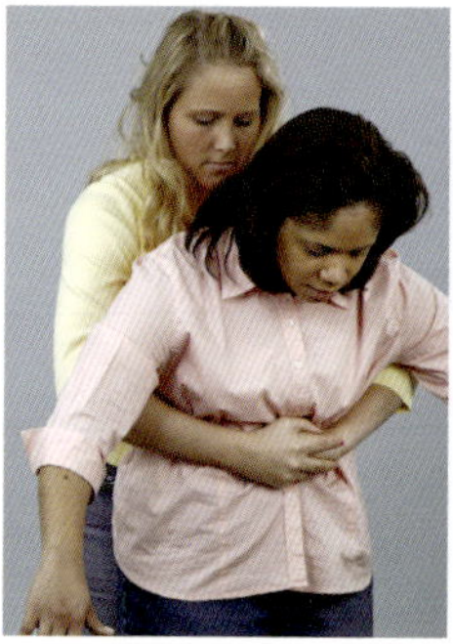

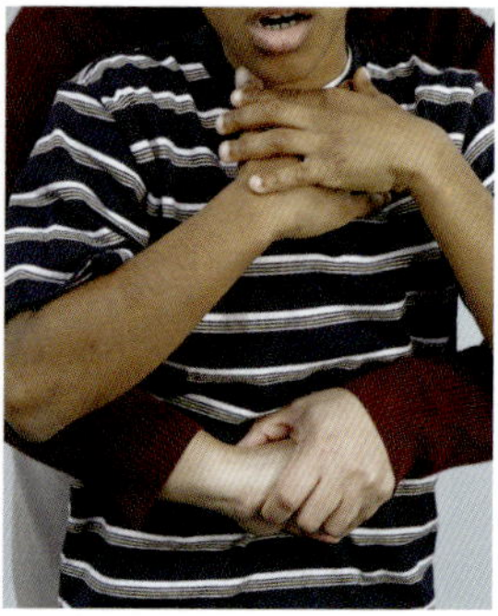

Repeat back blows and abdominal thrusts until—
- Object is forced out and person breathes or coughs forcefully on his or her own; or
- Person becomes unconscious.

If person becomes unconscious—
- Call 9-1-1 if you have not already done so, and give care for Unconscious Choking Adult or Unconscious Choking Child. (Go to UNCONSCIOUS CHOKING—ADULT, page 19, or UNCONSCIOUS CHOKING—CHILD, page 21.)

CONSCIOUS CHOKING—INFANT (UNDER AGE 1)

What to look for:

- Cannot cough, cry or breathe
- Coughing weakly or making high-pitched sounds

What to do:

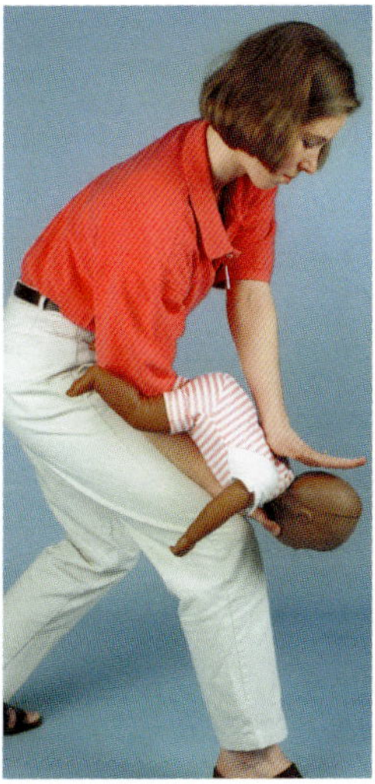

- CHECK the scene and the infant.
- If coughing forcefully, do not give back blows to the infant.
- Send someone to CALL 9-1-1 or the local emergency number.
- Get permission to give care from parent or guardian, if present.
- Give 5 back blows (between the shoulder blades) and 5 chest thrusts.

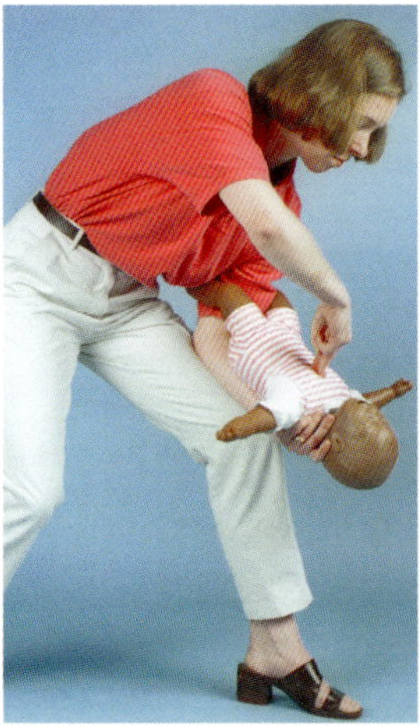

(Hold infant's head and neck securely when giving back blows and chest thrusts.) Repeat back blows and chest thrusts until—

- The object is forced out and the infant breathes or coughs forcefully on its own; or
- The infant becomes unconscious.

If infant becomes unconscious—

- CALL 9-1-1 if you have not already done so, and give care for Unconscious Choking Infant. (Go to UNCONSCIOUS CHOKING—INFANT, page 23.)

UNCONSCIOUS CHOKING—ADULT

What to look for:

- Unable to make the chest clearly rise when giving rescue breaths.

What to do:

- Call or send someone to CALL 9-1-1 or the local emergency number if you have not already done so.
- Tilt the head and lift the chin, then pinch the nose shut.
- Make a seal over person's mouth.
- Give 2 rescue breaths.

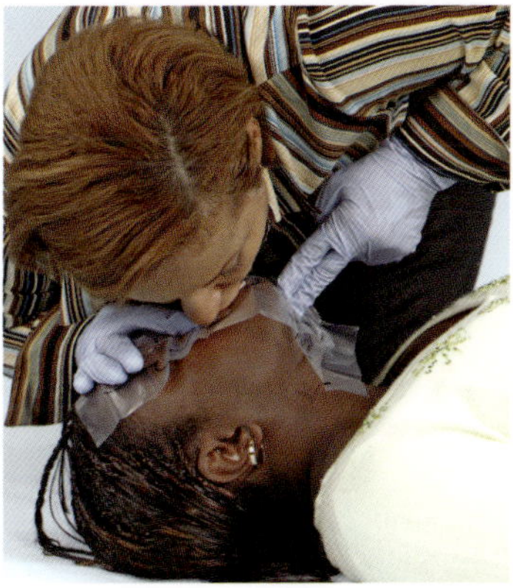

If breaths do not go in—

- Tilt head farther back.
- Try 2 rescue breaths again.

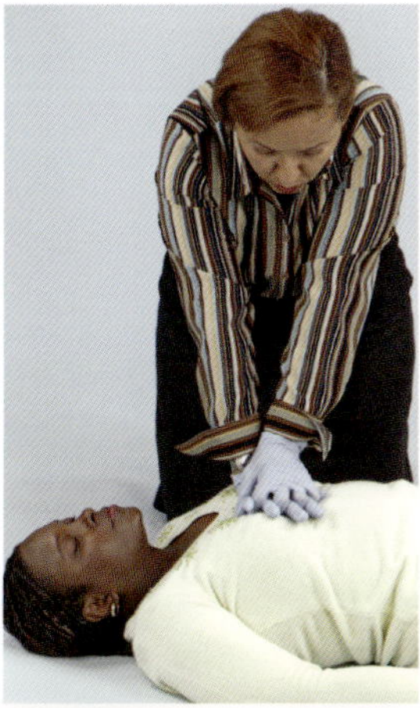

If chest does not rise—

- Remove CPR breathing barrier, if using one.
- Give 30 chest compressions.

- Look for an object.

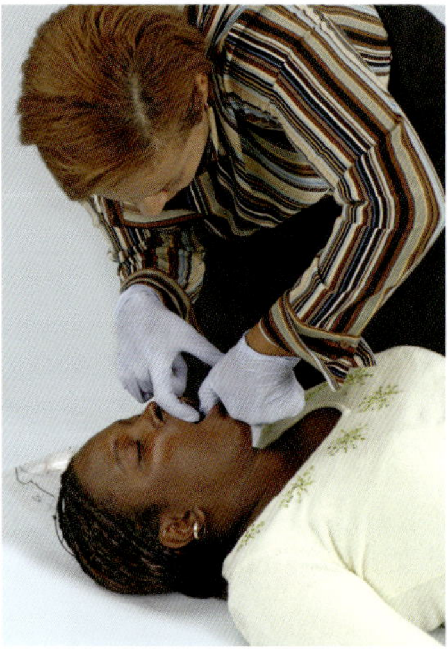

- Remove if one is seen.
- Try 2 rescue breaths.

If breaths still do not go in—

- Continue sets of 30 compressions, followed by looking for object/removal and giving 2 rescue breaths until—
  - The chest clearly rises with rescue breaths.
  - The person starts breathing.
  - EMS arrives.
  - Another trained responder takes over.
  - You are too exhausted to continue.
  - The scene becomes unsafe.

If breaths go in—

- Check for signs of life.
- Give care based on conditions found. (Go to TABLE OF CONTENTS, page iii.)

UNCONSCIOUS CHOKING—CHILD (AGES 1-12)

What to look for:

- Unable to make the chest clearly rise when giving rescue breaths.

What to do:

- Call or send someone to CALL 9-1-1 or the local emergency number if you have not already done so.
- If alone, give 2 minutes of care before calling.
- Tilt the head and lift the chin, then pinch the nose shut.
- Make a seal over child's mouth.
- Give 2 rescue breaths.

If breaths do not go in—

- Retilt child's head down and back to neutral position.
- Try 2 rescue breaths again.

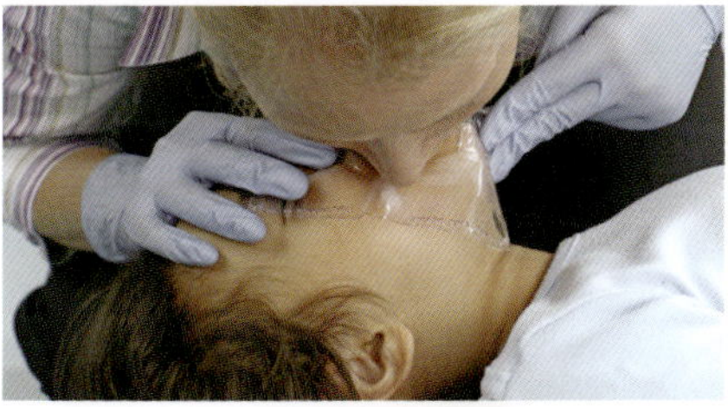

If chest does not rise—

- Remove CPR breathing barrier, if using one.
- Give 30 chest compressions.

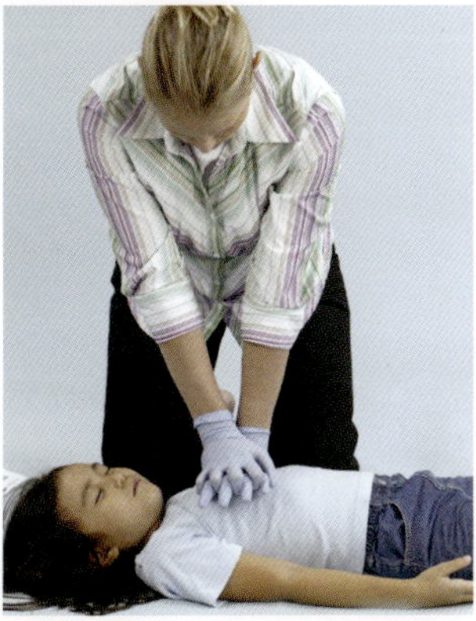

- Look for an object.
- Remove with finger if one is seen.

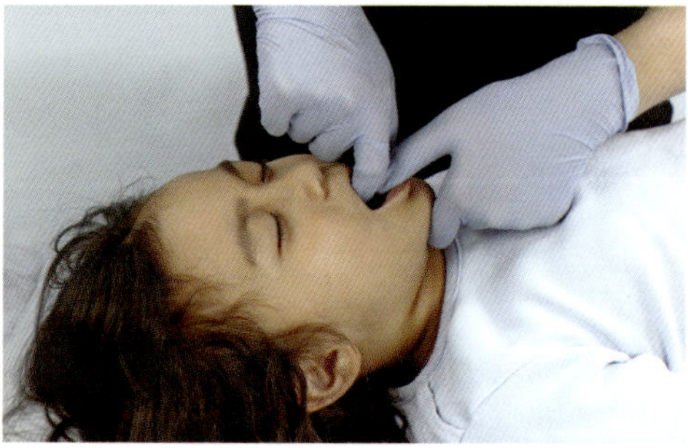

- Try 2 rescue breaths.

If breaths still do not go in—

- Continue sets of 30 compressions, followed by look for object/removal and 2 rescue breaths until—
  - Chest clearly rises with rescue breaths.
  - The child starts breathing.
  - EMS arrives.
  - Another trained responder takes over.
  - You are too exhausted to continue.
  - The scene becomes unsafe.

If breaths go in—

- Check for signs of life.
- Give care based on conditions found. (Go to TABLE OF CONTENTS, page iii.)

UNCONSCIOUS CHOKING—INFANT (UNDER AGE 1)

What to look for:

- Unable to make the chest clearly rise when giving rescue breaths.

What to do:

- Call or send someone to CALL 9-1-1 or the local emergency number, if you have not already done so.
- If alone, give 2 minutes of care before calling.
- Tilt the head and lift the chin.
- Make a seal over infant's mouth and nose.
- Give 2 rescue breaths.

If breaths do not go in—

- Retilt infant's head down and back to neutral position.
- Try 2 rescue breaths again.

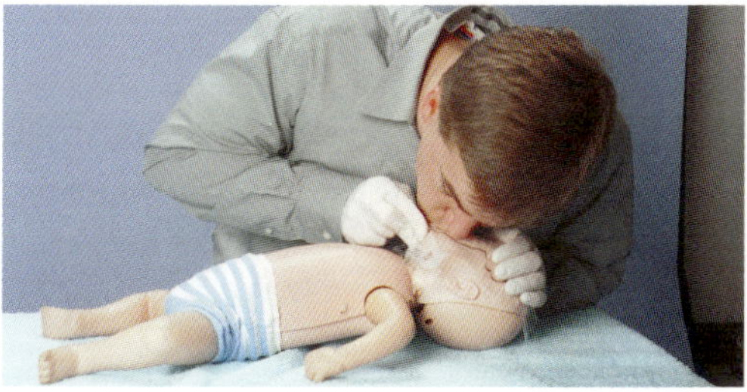

If chest does not rise—

- Remove CPR breathing barrier, if using one.
- Give 30 chest compressions.

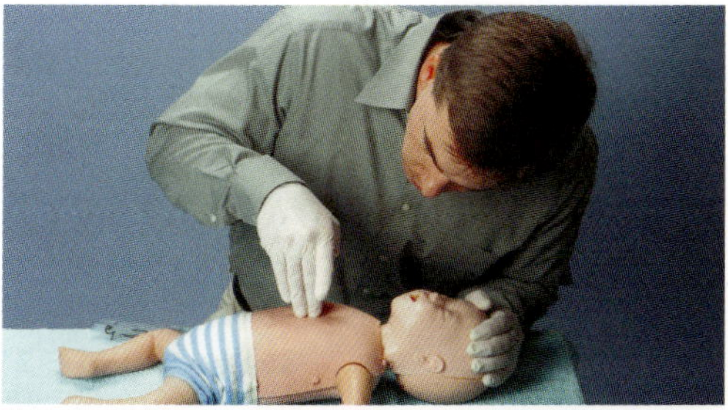

- Look for an object.
- Remove if one is seen.

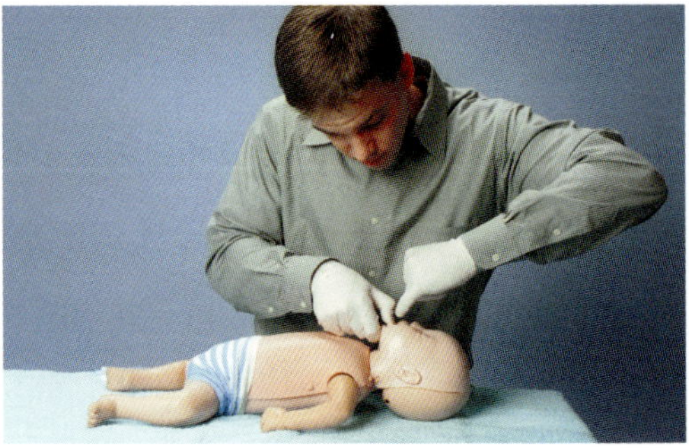

- Try 2 rescue breaths.

If breaths still do not go in—
- Continue sets of 30 compressions, followed by look for object/removal and 2 rescue breaths until—
  - Chest clearly rises with rescue breaths.
  - The infant starts breathing.
  - EMS arrives and takes over.
  - Another trained responder takes over.
  - You are too exhausted to continue.
  - The scene becomes unsafe.

If breaths go in—
- Check for signs of life.
- Give care based on conditions found. (Go to TABLE OF CONTENTS, page iii.)

CUTS, SCRAPES AND BLEEDING

When to Call 9-1-1 or the Local Emergency Number

- Bleeding that cannot be stopped
- Wounds that show muscle or bone, involve joints, are deep or involve hands or feet
- Large wounds
- Large or deeply embedded objects in the wound
- Human or animal bites
- Any wound on the face
- Skin or body parts that have been partially or completely torn away

What to do:

- CHECK the scene and the person.
- Get permission to give care.
- Cover the wound with a sterile dressing and apply direct pressure. Avoid touching blood or body fluids; wear disposable gloves FIRST AID or use a barrier.
- Cover dressing with a bandage FIRST AID to maintain pressure.

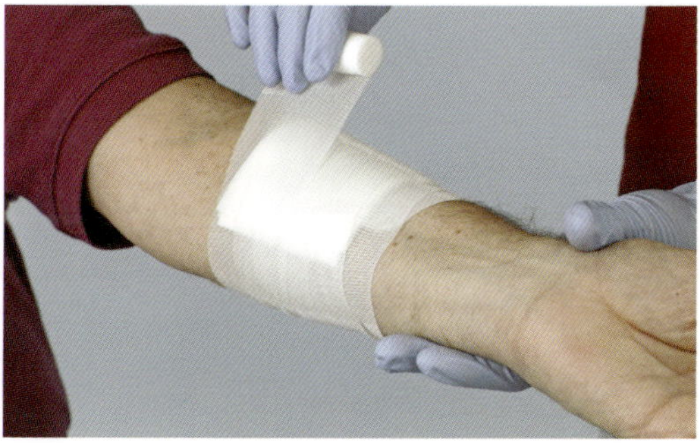

- Wash hands immediately after giving care even if you use gloves.

If bleeding does not stop—
- Apply additional dressings and bandage FIRST AID to maintain pressure.
- Call or have someone else CALL 9-1-1 or the local emergency number.
- Care for shock.

MINOR WOUND CARE

What to do:
- CHECK the scene and the person.
- Get permission to give care.
- Using a barrier, apply direct pressure to control bleeding.
- Wash the wound with soap and water. Rinse for about 5 minutes with clean running tap water.
- Apply a triple antibiotic ointment FIRST AID or cream if the person has no known allergies or sensitivities to the medication.
- Cover the wound with a sterile dressing and bandage FIRST AID.

NOSEBLEED

What to do:
- CHECK the scene and the person.
- Get permission to give care.
- Have person lean slightly forward.
- Pinch the nose shut for about 10 minutes.
- Apply a non-chemical ice pack to the bridge of the nose.

If bleeding does not stop—
- Apply pressure on upper lip just beneath nose.
- Seek medical care.

DIABETIC EMERGENCY

Diabetics sometimes become ill because there is too much or too little sugar in their blood. In either case, giving sugar will not cause additional harm.

What to do:

- CHECK the scene and the person.
- Get permission to give care.
- If person is conscious and can safely swallow food or fluids and is a known diabetic, give sugar (fruit juices, nondiet soft drinks, table sugar).
- If person is not feeling better in about 5 minutes, CALL 9-1-1 or the local emergency number.
- If person is unconscious—
  - DO NOT GIVE ANYTHING TO EAT OR DRINK.
  - Send someone to CALL 9-1-1 or the local emergency number.
  - CHECK the person, then CARE for the conditions you find. (Go to TABLE OF CONTENTS, page iii.)

DROWNING

What to do:

- Send someone to CALL 9-1-1 or the local emergency number.
- Attempt to rescue by reaching or throwing an object that floats to the person. DO NOT ATTEMPT A SWIMMING RESCUE UNLESS YOU HAVE PROPER EQUIPMENT AND ARE TRAINED TO DO SO.

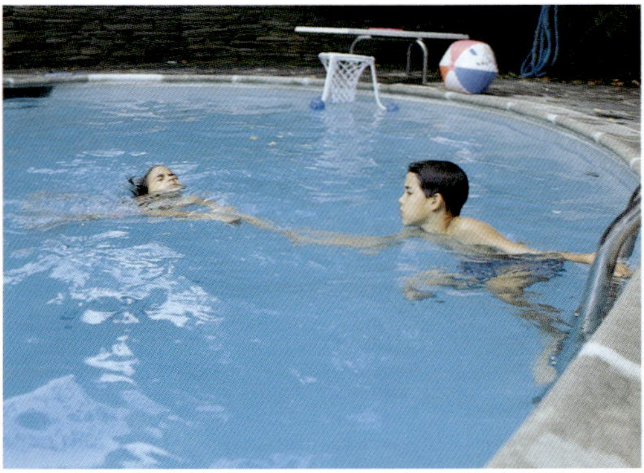

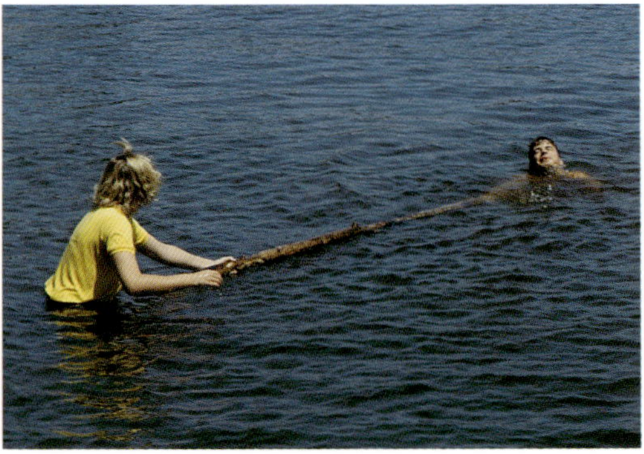

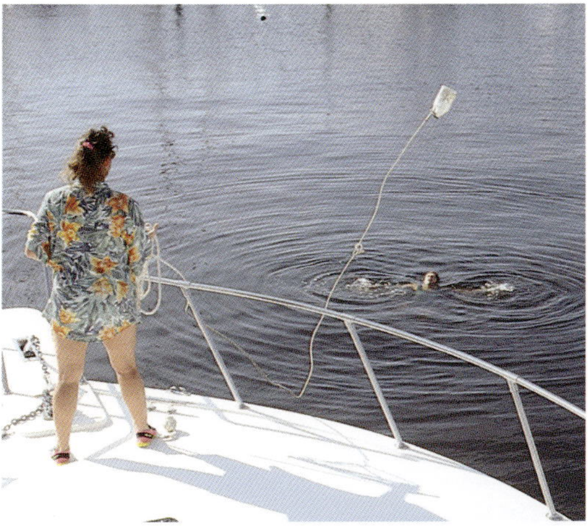

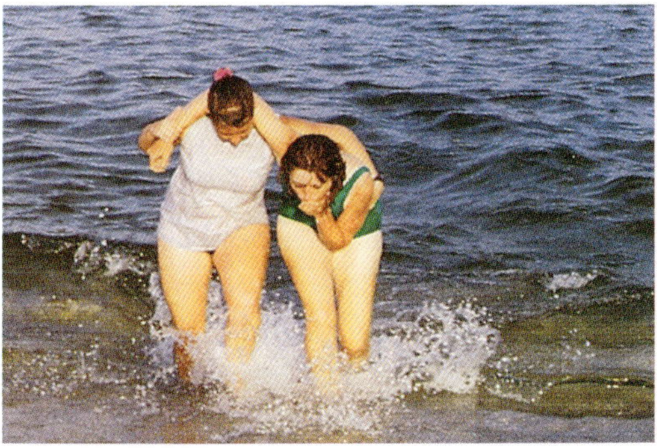

Once the person is out of the water—

- Tilt the head back, lift chin and CHECK for signs of life.

If no breathing—

- Give 2 rescue breaths.

If breaths go in—

- Give CPR. (Go to CPR, page 37.)

If breaths do not go in—

- Retilt the head and try 2 breaths again. (Go to UNCONSCIOUS CHOKING, page 19.)

EMBEDDED OBJECT

What to look for:

- Pain
- Visible object with open wound
- Bleeding

What to do:

- CHECK the scene and the person.
- Send someone to CALL 9-1-1 or the local emergency number.
- Get permission to give care.
- DO NOT REMOVE OBJECT.
- Place bulky dressings around the object to support object in place.
- Use a roller bandage FIRST AID to secure the dressing in place.

FAINTING

Fainting is not usually harmful and the person will usually recover quickly.

What to do:

- Send someone to CALL 9-1-1 or the local emergency number.
- Lower the person to the ground or other flat surface and position on his or her back.
- Elevate legs 8 to 12 inches if injury is not suspected.
- Loosen any tight clothing.
- Check breathing.
- Do not give anything to eat or drink.

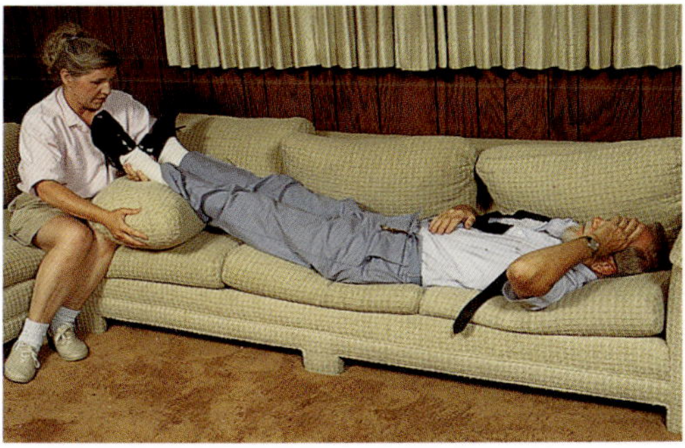

FROSTBITE AND HYPOTHERMIA

FROSTBITE

What to look for:

- Lack of feeling in the affected area.
- Skin appears waxy, is cold to the touch or discolored (flushed, white, gray, yellow or blue).

What to do:

- CHECK the scene and the person.
- Send someone to CALL 9-1-1 or the local emergency number.
- Try to remove jewelry and wet clothing.
- Handle the frostbitten area gently. DO NOT rub the affected area.
- Warm gently by soaking affected area in warm water (100° F to 105° F) until normal color returns and the frostbitten part feels warm.

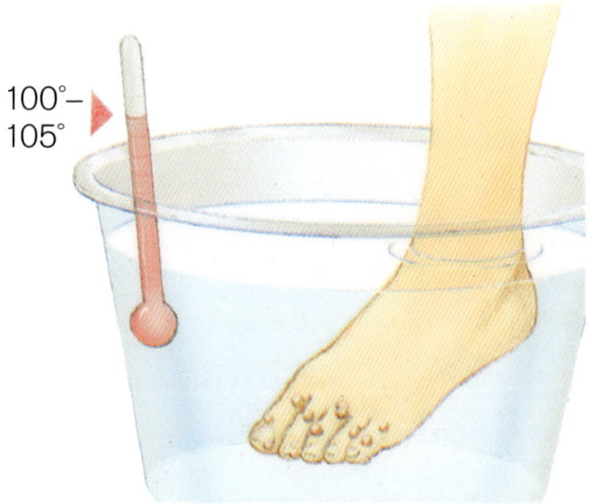

- Loosely bandage area with dry, sterile dressing.

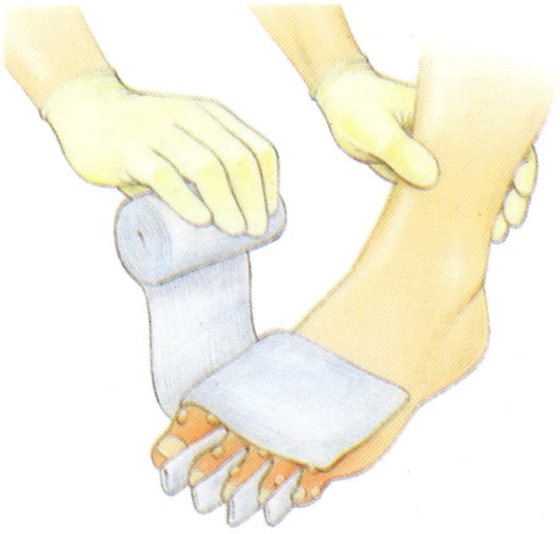

- If fingers or toes are frostbitten, place dry, sterile gauze between them to keep them separated.
- Avoid breaking any blisters.

HYPOTHERMIA

What to look for:

- Shivering, numbness, glassy stare
- Apathy, weakness, impaired judgment
- Loss of consciousness

What to do:

- CHECK the scene and the person.
- Send someone to CALL 9-1-1 or the local emergency number.
- Care for life-threatening conditions. (Go to LIFE-THREATENING EMERGENCIES, page viii.)
- GENTLY move the person to a warm place.
- Remove any wet clothing and dry the person.
- Warm the person gradually by wrapping in blankets FIRST AID or putting dry clothing on the person.
- If the person is alert, give warm liquids that *do not* contain alcohol or caffeine.
- DO NOT WARM PERSON TOO QUICKLY, such as immersing him or her in warm water. Rapid warming can cause dangerous heart rhythms.

FIRST AID CONDITIONS H TO Z

FIRST AID H-Z

HEAD, NECK AND BACK INJURIES

What to look for:

- Person was involved in a motor-vehicle crash.
- Person was injured as a result of a fall from greater than a standing height.
- Person complains of neck or back pain.
- Person feels tingling or weakness in extremities.
- Person is not fully alert.
- Person appears to be intoxicated.
- Person appears to be frail or over age 65.

What to do:

- CHECK the scene and the person.
- Get permission to give care.
- CALL 9-1-1 or the local emergency number.
- Minimize movement.
- Manually support the person's head as found.

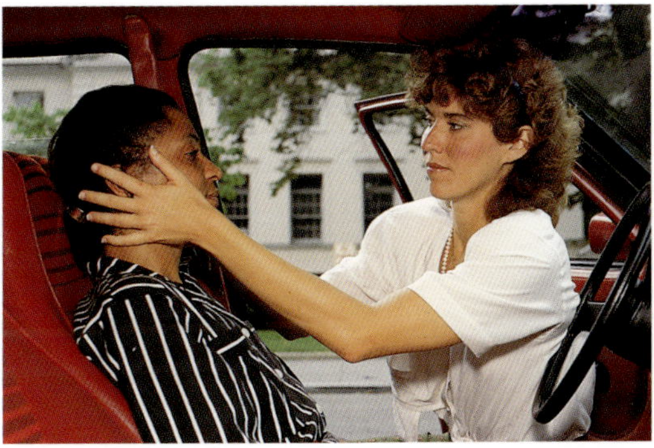

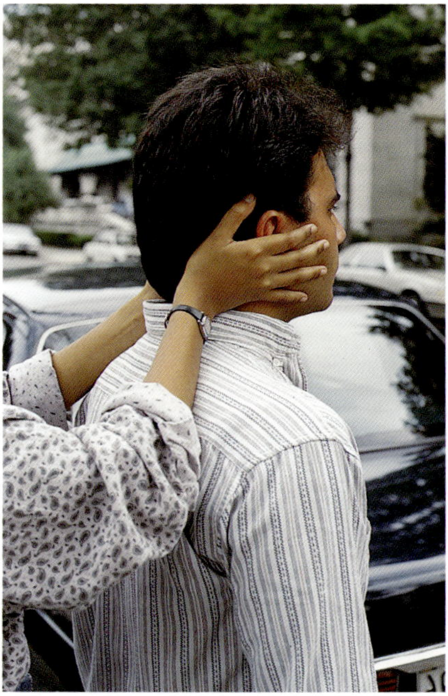

- If the head is sharply turned to one side, DO NOT move it.

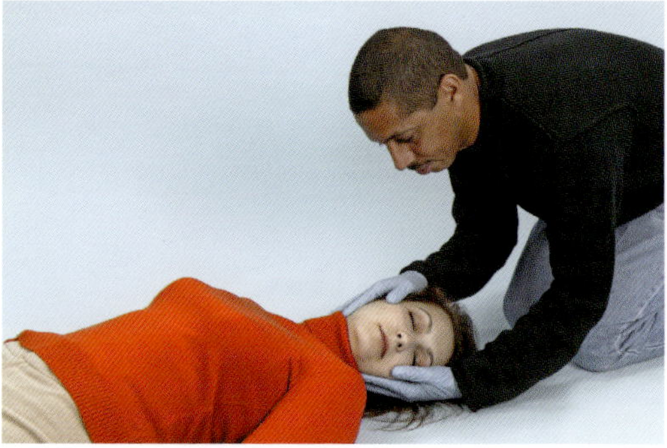

- Support the head in the position found.

HEART ATTACK/CARDIAC ARREST/ CPR/AED

The American Red Cross strongly recommends that you take a course in CPR to learn how to perform CPR and use an AED.

HEART ATTACK

What to look for:

- Persistent chest pain or discomfort lasting more than 3 to 5 minutes or that goes away and comes back
  - May spread to shoulder, arm, back, neck or jaw
- Shortness of breath or trouble breathing
- Nausea or vomiting
- Sweating or changes in skin appearance
- Dizziness, light-headedness or fainting
- May complain of heartburn or indigestion
  - These signals are more likely to occur in women, the elderly and diabetics.
- Denial that anything serious is wrong

What to do:

- CHECK the scene and the person.
- Send someone to CALL 9-1-1 or the local emergency number.
- Have the person stop activity and rest.
- Help the person rest in a comfortable position. A sitting position may make breathing easier.
- Loosen restrictive clothing.
- Assist with prescribed medication.
- Offer aspirin FIRST AID if medically appropriate.

Aspirin administration assistance:

- Never delay calling 9-1-1 or the local emergency number to administer aspirin.
- Ask if the person is able to take medicine by the mouth. If yes, then ask if he or she—
  - Is allergic to aspirin.
  - Has a stomach ulcer or stomach disease.
  - Is taking any blood thinners such as Coumadin™ or warfarin.
  - Has been told by a physician not to take aspirin.
- If the person answers no to all of the above questions, you may offer 2 chewable (162 mg) baby aspirin, or 1 adult aspirin FIRST AID (325 mg) with a small amount of water.
- Monitor signs of life closely.
- Be prepared to give CPR if the person loses consciousness and shows no signs of life.
- Be prepared to use an AED.

CARDIAC ARREST—ADULT

What to look for:

- Does not respond (unconscious)
- No signs of life (movement or breathing)

What to do:

- CHECK the scene and the person.
- Call or send someone to CALL 9-1-1 or the local emergency number.
- CHECK for signs of life for no more than 10 seconds.
- Give 2 rescue breaths.

CPR—ADULT

If no signs of life—

- Begin **CPR—Adult.**
- If you are unwilling, unable or untrained on full CPR, you should give continuous chest compressions once EMS system has been activated.

1. Compress chest 30 times.

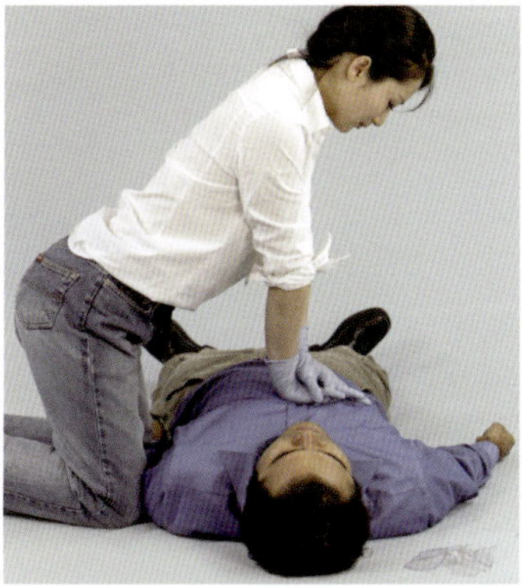

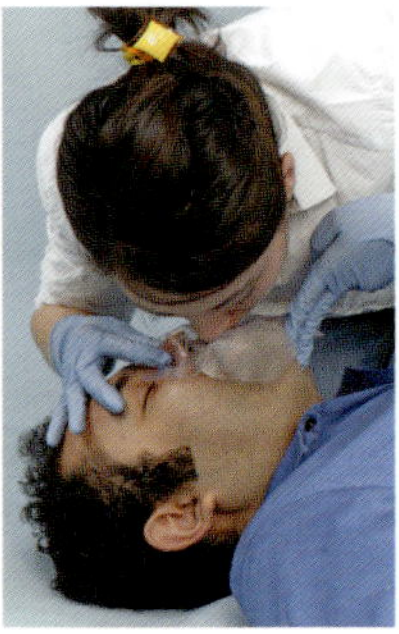

2. Give 2 rescue breaths.
   - Tilt the head and lift the chin, then pinch the nose shut.
   - Make seal over person's mouth.
   - Give 2 rescue breaths.
3. Continue cycles of 30 compressions and 2 breaths until—
   - The scene becomes unsafe.
   - You find a sign of life.
   - An AED is ready to use.
   - You are too exhausted to continue.
   - Another trained responder arrives and takes over.

If breaths do not go in—
- Go to UNCONSCIOUS CHOKING—ADULT, page 19.

Use a CPR breathing barrier FIRST AID if one is available.

AED—ADULT
(Ages 8 and older)

What to do:

If an AED is ready to use—

- Turn on the AED.

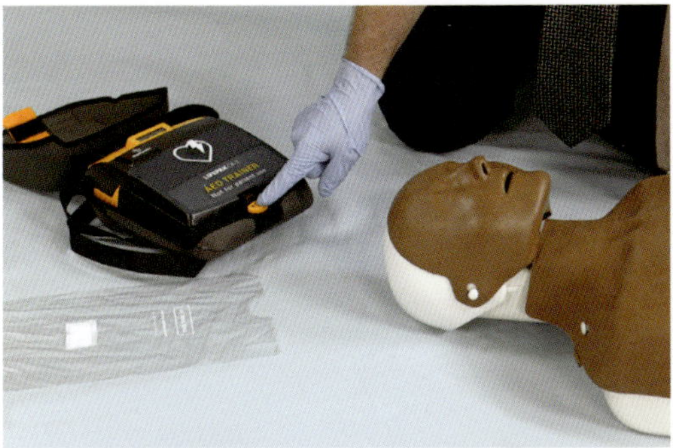

- Wipe chest dry.

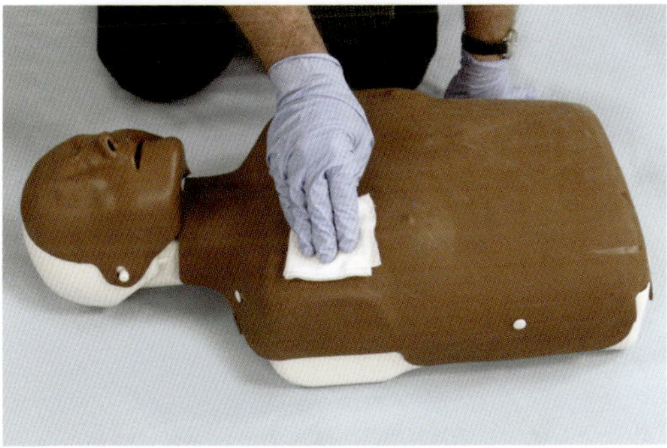

• Attach pads to bare chest.

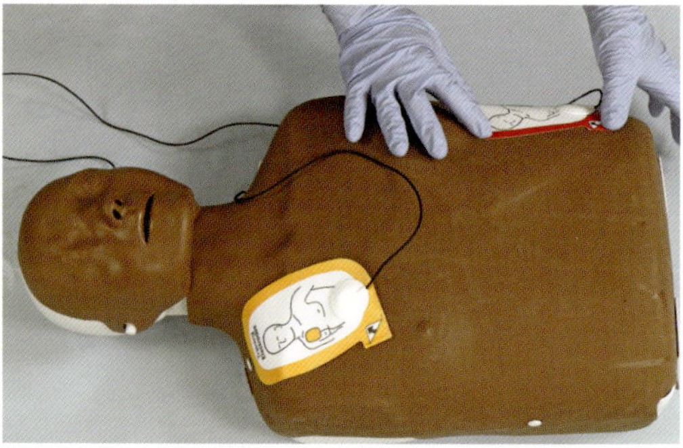

• Plug in the connector, if necessary.

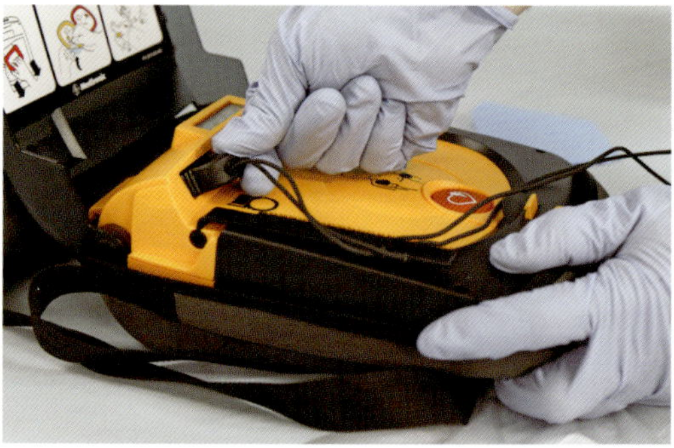

• Make sure no one, including you, is touching the person. Tell everyone to "stand clear."

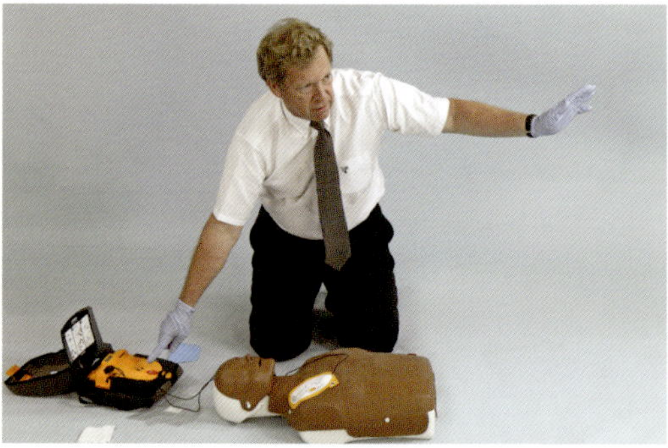

• Push the "analyze" button, if necessary. Let the AED analyze the heart rhythm.

If the AED advises you to shock the person—

- Make sure no one, including you, is touching the person.
- Tell everyone to "stand clear."
- Push the "shock" button if necessary.

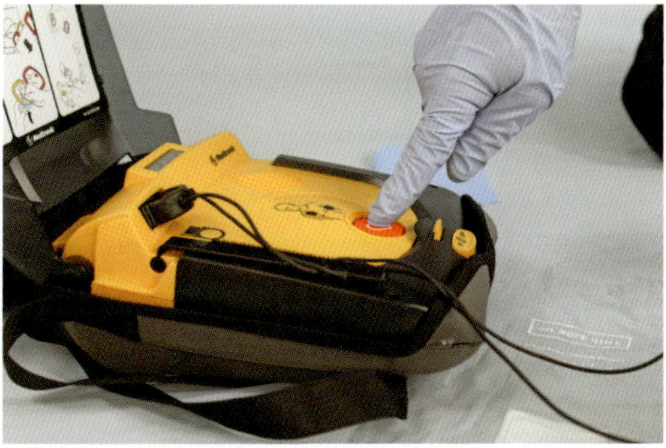

After shock is delivered—

- Give 5 cycles or about 2 minutes of CPR.
- Let the AED reanalyze.
- If the AED says "no shock advised," give 5 cycles or about 2 minutes of CPR.

CARDIAC ARREST—CHILD

What to look for:

- Does not respond (unconscious)
- No signs of life (movement or breathing)

What to do:

- CHECK the scene and the child.
- Send someone to CALL 9-1-1 or the local emergency number.
- If you are alone, give 2 minutes of care before calling.
- CHECK for signs of life for no more than 10 seconds.
- Give 2 rescue breaths.

CPR—CHILD

If no signs of life—

- Begin **CPR—Child.**
- If you are unwilling, unable or untrained on full CPR, you should give continuous chest compressions once EMS system has been activated.

1. Compress chest 30 times.

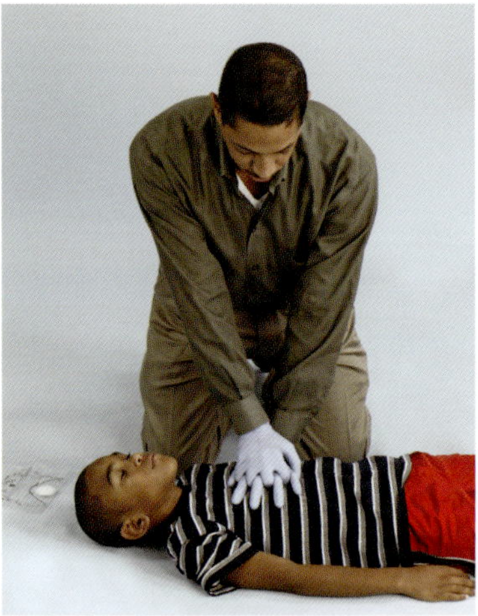

2. Give 2 rescue breaths.

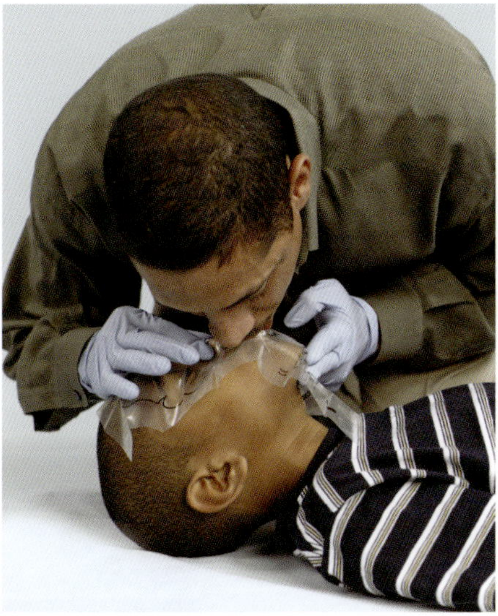

- Tilt the head and lift the chin, then pinch the nose shut.
- Make seal over child's mouth.
- Give 2 rescue breaths.

3. Continue cycles of 30 compressions and 2 breaths until—
   - The scene becomes unsafe.
   - You find a sign of life.
   - An AED is ready to use.
   - You are too exhausted to continue.
   - Another trained responder arrives and takes over.

If breaths do not go in—
- Go to UNCONSCIOUS CHOKING—CHILD, page 21.

Use a CPR breathing barrier FIRST AID if one is available.

AED—CHILD
(Ages 1 to 8 or less than 55 pounds)

What to do:

If an AED is ready to use—

- Turn on the AED.

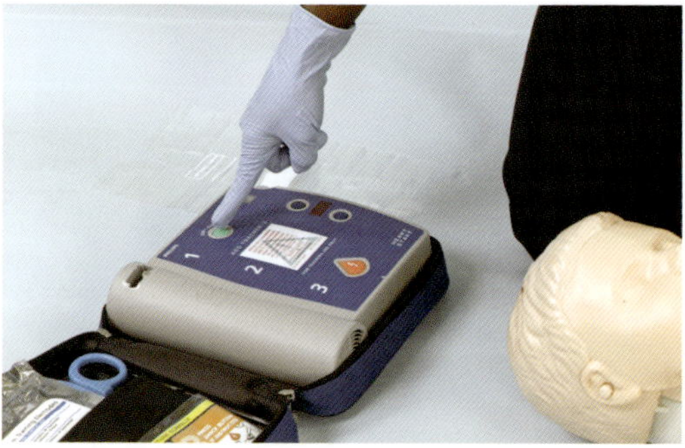

- Wipe chest dry.

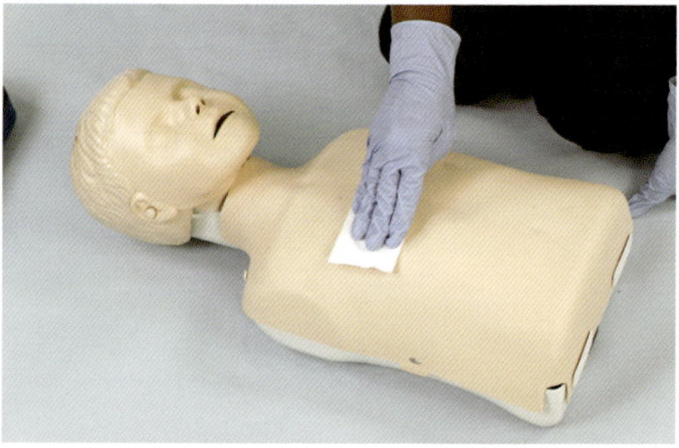

- Attach pediatric pads to child's bare chest.

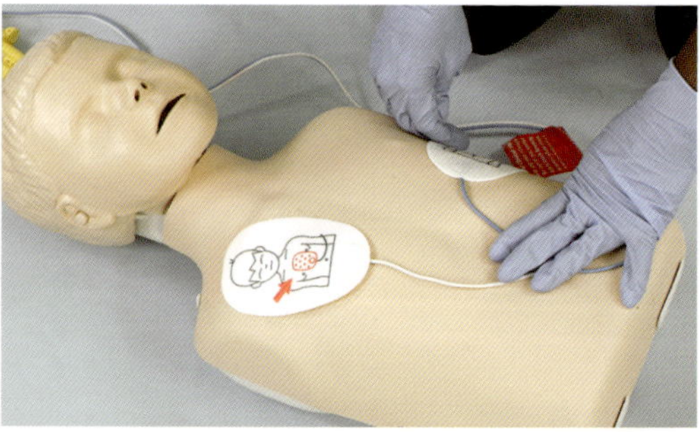

- If pads risk touching each other, use front/back pad placement.

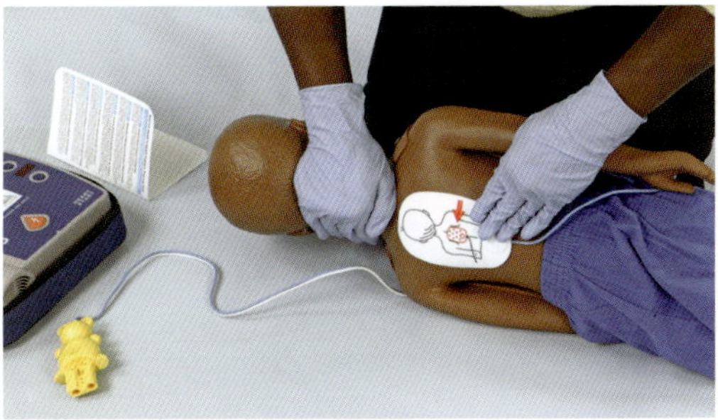

- Plug in the connector, if necessary.

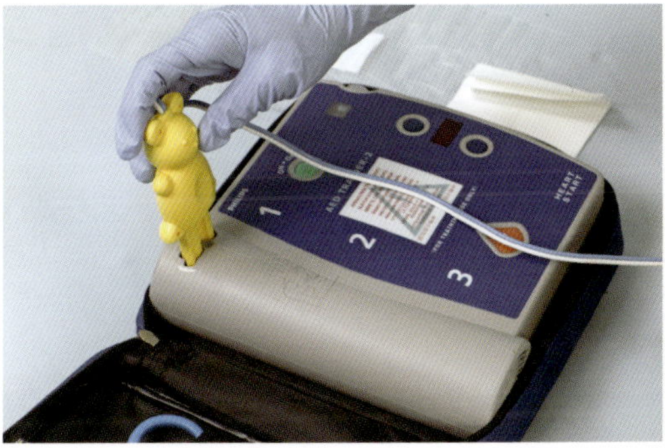

- Make sure no one, including you, is touching the child. Tell everyone to "stand clear."

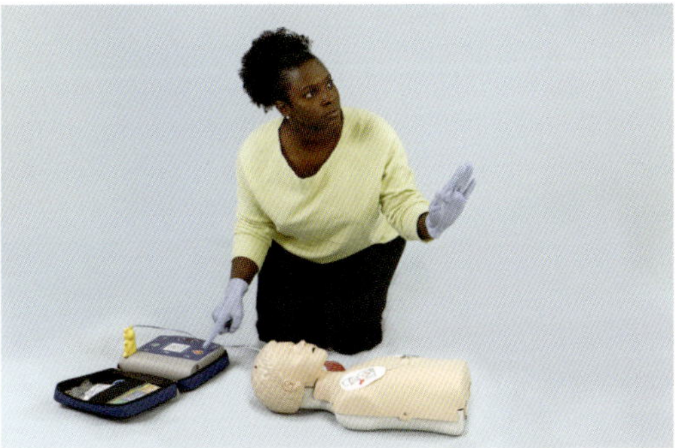

- Push the "analyze" button, if necessary. Let the AED analyze the child's heart rhythm.

If the AED advises you to shock the child—
- Make sure no one, including you, is touching the child.
- Tell everyone to "stand clear."
- Push the "shock" button, if necessary.

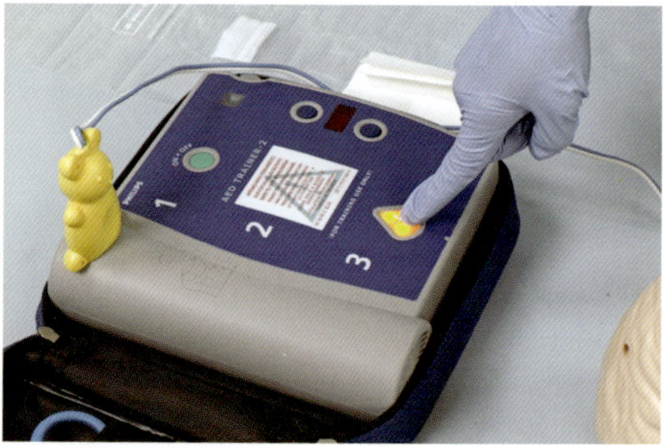

After shock is delivered—
- Give 5 cycles or about 2 minutes of CPR.
- Let the AED reanalyze.
- If the AED says "no shock advised," give 5 cycles or about 2 minutes of CPR.

CARDIAC ARREST—INFANT

What to look for:

- Does not respond (unconscious)
- No signs of life (movement and breathing)

What to do:

- CHECK the scene and the infant.
- Send someone to CALL 9-1-1 or the local emergency number.
- If alone, give 2 minutes of care before calling.
- CHECK for signs of life for no more than 10 seconds.
- Give 2 rescue breaths.

CPR—INFANT

If no signs of life—

- Begin **CPR—Infant.**
- If you are unwilling, unable or untrained on full CPR, you should give continuous chest compressions once EMS system has been activated.

1. Compress chest 30 times.

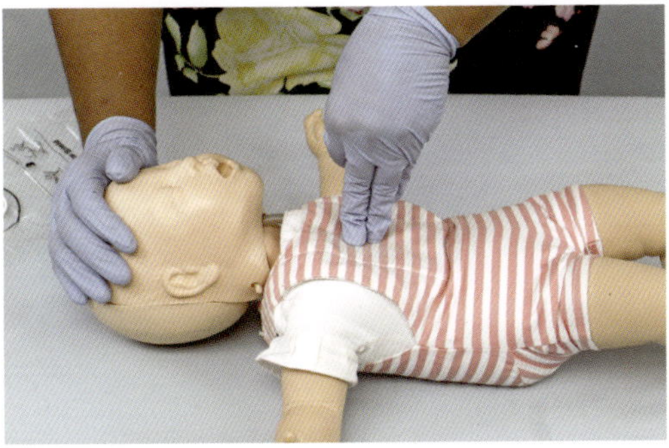

2. Give 2 rescue breaths.

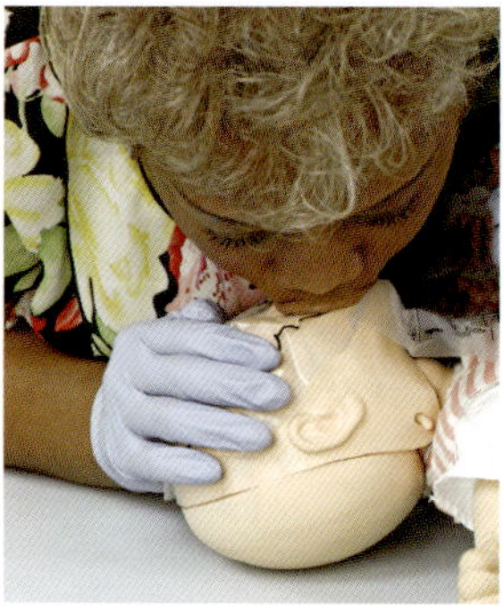

   - Tilt the head and lift the chin.
   - Make seal over infant's mouth and nose.
   - Give 2 rescue breaths.
3. Continue cycles of 30 compressions and 2 breaths until—
   - The scene becomes unsafe.
   - You find a sign of life.
   - You are too exhausted to continue.
   - Another trained responder arrives and takes over.

If breaths do not go in—

- Go to UNCONSCIOUS CHOKING—INFANT, page 23.

Use a CPR breathing barrier FIRST AID if one is available.

HEAT-RELATED EMERGENCIES

HEAT CRAMPS

What to look for:

- Painful muscle spasms, usually in the legs and abdomen

What to do:

- CHECK the scene and the person.
- Get permission to give care.
- Have person rest in a cool place.
- If the person is conscious, give small amounts of cool water or a commercial sports drink.
- Lightly stretch and gently massage the muscle.
- DO NOT GIVE SALT TABLETS.
- Watch for signals of heat illness.

HEAT EXHAUSTION (Early Stages)

What to look for:

- Cool, moist, pale or flushed skin
- Headache, nausea, dizziness
- Weakness, exhaustion
- Heavy sweating

HEAT STROKE (Late Stages)

What to look for:

- Red, hot, dry skin
- Changes in level of consciousness
- Rapid, weak pulse
- Rapid, shallow breathing
- Vomiting

What to do:

- Move person to a cool place.
- Loosen tight or remove perspiration-soaked clothing.
- Apply cool, wet cloths to the skin or mist with cool water and fan the person.
- If conscious, give small amounts of cool water to drink.

If person does not improve quickly, refuses water, vomits, loses consciousness or shows signs of heat stroke (late stages)—

- Send someone to CALL 9-1-1 or the local emergency number and place person on his or her side.
- Continue to cool by placing ice or cold packs on person's wrists, ankles, groin and neck and in armpits.
- If the person becomes unconscious, be prepared to give CPR, if necessary. (Go to CPR, page 37.)

MUSCLE, BONE AND JOINT INJURIES

SPLINTING

Splinting is a method used to keep an injured body part from moving. It can also help reduce pain, making the injured person more comfortable.

- Splint **only** if the person must be moved or transported and if you can do so without causing more pain and discomfort to the person.
- Splint an injury in the position you find it.
- Splint the joints above and below an injured bone.
- Splint the bones above and below an injured joint.
- Check for feeling, warmth and color of the skin below the site of injury both before and after splinting.
- If the injury appears serious, or the person cannot be safely transported, CALL 9-1-1 or the local emergency number.

What to do:

For a leg injury—

- CHECK the scene and the person.
- Get permission to give care.
- Immobilize the injured leg by binding it to the uninjured leg with a triangular bandage FIRST AID.

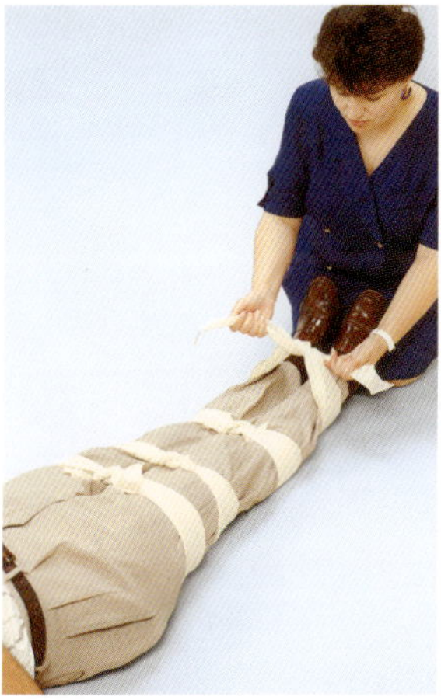

For fractured ribs—

- CHECK the scene and the person.
- Get permission to give care.
- Place a pillow or folded blanket FIRST AID between the injured ribs and the arm.

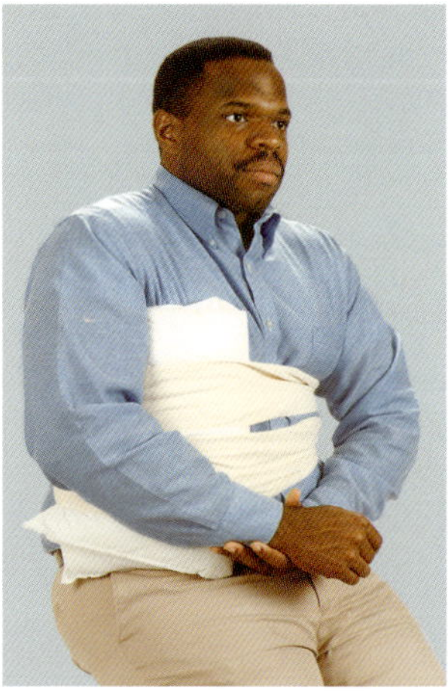

- Bind the arm to the body to help support the injured area.

For ankle and foot injuries—

- CHECK the scene and the person.
- Get permission to give care.
- Immobilize the ankle and foot by using a soft splint—a pillow or blanket FIRST AID.

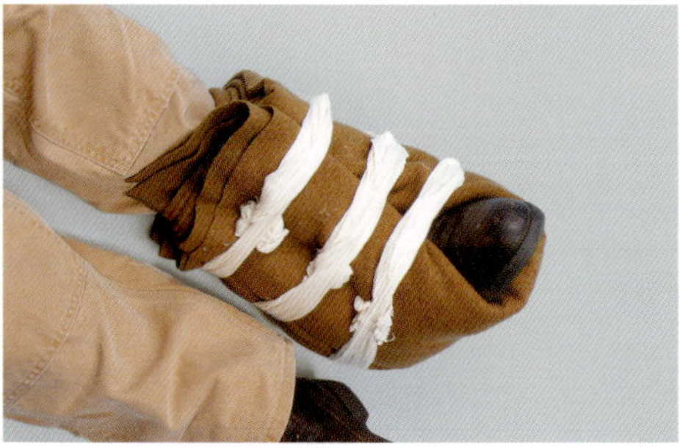

- Do not remove the person's shoe.

For hand and finger injuries—

- CHECK the scene and the person.
- Get permission to give care.
- If you suspect that the finger is broken or dislocated, tape the injured finger to a finger next to it.

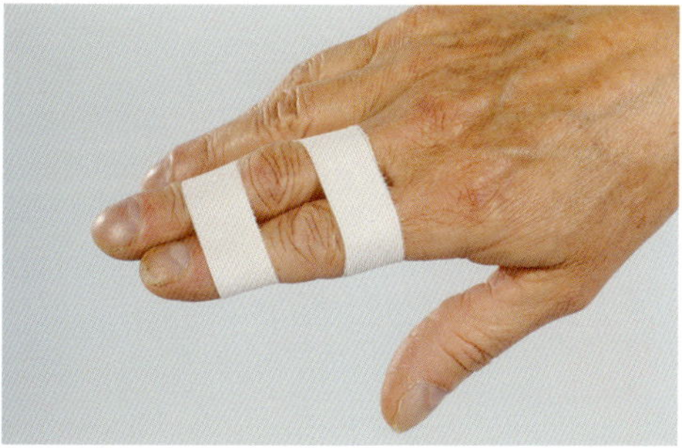

POISONING

What to look for:

- Trouble breathing
- Nausea, vomiting, diarrhea
- Chest or abdominal pain
- Sweating, changes in consciousness, seizures
- Burns around the lips or tongue, or on the skin
- Open or spilled containers; open medicine cabinet
- Overturned or damaged plant
- Unusual odors, flames, smoke
- Headache
- Dizziness

What to do:

- CHECK the scene to make sure it is safe to approach and gather clues about what happened.
- Look for any containers.
- If necessary, move the person to safety, away from the source of the poison.
- CHECK the person's level of consciousness and signs of life (movement and breathing).
- If you suspect that a person is showing signals of poisoning, call the National Poison Control Center (PCC) at 800-222-1222.
- CARE for any life-threatening conditions, if found, and CALL 9-1-1 or the local emergency number. (Go to LIFE-THREATENING EMERGENCIES, page viii.)
- DO NOT give the person anything to eat or drink unless directed to do so by PCC or EMS.
- If you suspect someone has swallowed a poison, try to find out the type of poison, how much was taken and when it was taken.

- If the person vomits, position him or her on the side. Save a sample of the vomit if poison is unknown so that it can be identified at the hospital.

Poisonous Plants

- Get permission to give care.
- Immediately wash the affected area thoroughly with soap and water.
- If a rash or open sores develop, apply paste of baking soda and water several times a day to reduce discomfort.
- Apply lotions, such as Caladryl™, which may help soothe the area.
- If condition gets worse or affects large areas of the body or face, see a healthcare provider.
- Wash clothing exposed to plant oils.

SEIZURES

If you know the person has epilepsy, it is usually not necessary to CALL 9-1-1 or the local emergency number. Call if—

- The seizure lasts longer than 5 minutes or is repeated.
- The seizure follows a quick rise in the person's temperature.
- The person does not regain consciousness.
- The person is pregnant.
- The person is known to be a diabetic.
- The person is injured.
- The person shows other life-threatening conditions.
- The person has never had a seizure before.

What to do:

- CHECK the scene and the person.
- Send someone to CALL 9-1-1 or the local emergency number.
- Remove nearby objects that might cause injury.
- Protect the person's head by placing a folded towel or clothing beneath it.
- Do not hold or restrain person.
- Do not place anything between the person's teeth.
- Place the person on the side to drain fluids from mouth.
- When seizure is over, CHECK for breathing and injuries.
- Comfort and stay with person until he or she is fully conscious or EMS arrives and takes over.

SHOCK

What to look for:

The person—

- Is restless or irritable.
- Is nauseated or vomiting.
- Is experiencing an altered level of consciousness (e.g., is drowsy, confused or loses consciousness).
- Has pale, cool, moist skin.
- Has a blue tinge to lips and fingernails.
- Is breathing rapidly and has a rapid pulse.

What to do:

- CHECK the scene and the person.
- Send someone to CALL 9-1-1 or the local emergency number.
- Monitor the person's airway, breathing and circulation.
- Control any external bleeding.
- Keep the person from getting chilled or overheated.
- Elevate the legs about 8 to 12 inches if you do not suspect a head, neck or back injury or broken bones in the hips or legs.
- Comfort the person until EMS arrives.

STROKE

What to look for:

- Sudden body weakness or numbness, often on one side
- Sudden facial drooping or weakness on one side of the face
- Trouble speaking or being understood when speaking
- Trouble seeing in one or both eyes
- Sudden severe headache
- Dizziness, loss of balance
- Looking or feeling ill, abnormal behavior

What to do:

- CHECK the scene and the person.
- Send someone to CALL 9-1-1 or the local emergency number immediately.
- CARE for the specific conditions you find.
- If person is drooling or having difficulty swallowing, place person on the side to keep airway clear.

F.A.S.T. Recognition of Stroke

For a Stroke, Think F.A.S.T.

- **Face**—Weakness on one side of the face
  - Ask the person to smile; this will show if there is drooping or weakness in the muscles on one side of the face.

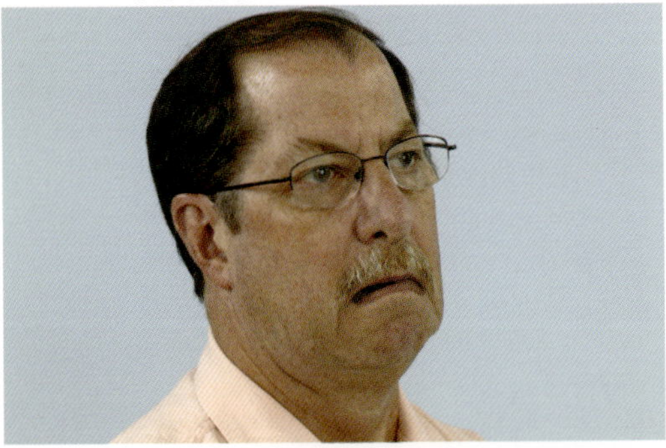

- **Arm—**Weakness or numbness in one arm
  - Ask the person to raise both arms to find out if there is weakness in one limb (both arms will not be raised to the same level).

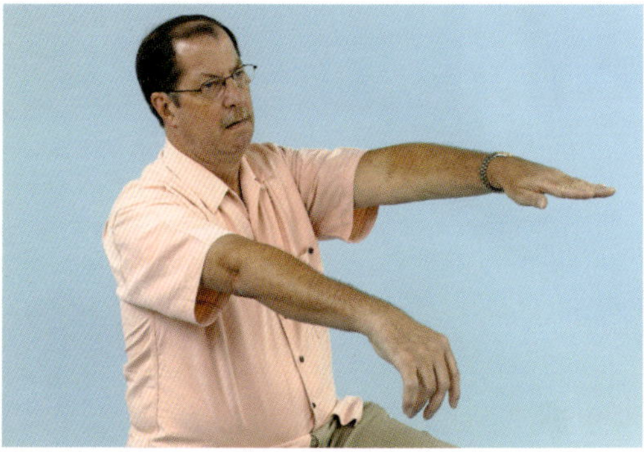

- **Speech—**Slurred speech or trouble getting the words out
  - Ask the person to say a simple sentence or phrase and listen for slurred or distorted speech (e.g., "Mary had a little lamb").
- **Time—**Time to CALL 9-1-1 if you see any of these signs
  - If the person has difficulty with any of these tasks or shows other signals of a stroke, note the time that the signals began and CALL 9-1-1 right away.

TOOTH (KNOCKED OUT)

What to do:

- Get permission to give care.
- If person is conscious and able to cooperate, rinse out the mouth with cold tap water, if available.
- Have person bite down on a rolled sterile dressing in the space left by the tooth to stop bleeding.
- Save any displaced teeth. Place them in milk, if possible, or cool water. Pick the tooth up by the crown (white part), not the root.
- Have person see a dentist immediately.

EMERGENCY PREPAREDNESS

EMERGENCY PREPAREDNESS

EMERGENCY PREPAREDNESS

EARTHQUAKES

Are You Ready for an Earthquake?

Here's what you can do to prepare for such an emergency.

Know What to Expect

Know your area's earthquake risk. If unsure, call your local American Red Cross chapter or emergency management office. Earthquakes strike suddenly, without warning, and recur in the same places. Earthquake-related injuries are often a result of collapsing walls, flying glass and falling objects, not the earthquake itself. Expect aftershocks, which can happen minutes, days, weeks and even months following an earthquake.

Reduce Potential Earthquake Damage By—

- Making sure your home is securely anchored to its foundation.
- Bolting and bracing water heaters and gas appliances to wall studs.
- Hanging heavy items such as pictures and mirrors away from beds and couches, and above places where people sleep or sit.
- Installing strong latches or bolts on cabinets.

Make a Plan

- Make sure your plan includes what to do if an earthquake occurs.
- Pick "safe places" in each room of your home, office or school under a sturdy table or desk or against an inside wall where nothing can fall on you.
- Practice drop, cover and hold on in each safe place.

- Keep a flashlight and sturdy shoes by each person's bed.
- Conduct periodic earthquake drills to ensure all family members know what to do if an earthquake happens.

For more information on making a plan, go to pages 76–78.

Get a Kit

For information on getting a kit for your family, go to pages 75–76.

During an Earthquake

- If you are inside when the shaking starts, you should drop, cover and hold on.
- If you are outdoors when the shaking starts, you should find a clear spot away from buildings and power lines, drop to the ground and stay there until the shaking stops.
- If you are in a vehicle, pull over to a clear location, stop and stay there with your seat belt fastened until the shaking stops.

RESIDENTIAL FIRES

Are You Ready for a Home Fire?

Here's what you can do to prepare for such an emergency.

Know What to Expect

All homes are at risk for fire. Contact your local American Red Cross chapter, fire department or emergency management office for more information about reducing your risk. Unlike other disasters, most fires can be prevented. The most effective way to protect yourself and your home from fire is to prevent a fire from starting.

Reduce Potential Fire Damage By—

- Identifying and eliminating fire hazards in your home.
- Installing and maintaining smoke alarms on every level of your home, outside sleeping areas and inside bedrooms, according to the manufacturer's instructions.
- Testing and dusting smoke alarms once a month.
- Changing the batteries in smoke alarms once a year.
- Replacing smoke alarms every 10 years.
- Installing residential fire sprinklers.

Increase Your Safety in Case of Fire By—

- Installing escape ladders for sleeping areas on the second or third floor.
- Using quick-release devices on barred windows and doors.
- Learning the emergency number for reporting a fire and practicing calling with young children.

Make a Plan

- Draw a floorplan of your home; mark two fire escape routes from each room.
- Select a safe outside meeting place for everyone to meet after escaping from a fire.
- Practice getting out of your home during the day and at night.
- Practice your escape plan at least twice a year.
- Make sure everyone in your home knows—
    - The two escape routes from each room.
    - To get out first, then call for help.
    - The location of the outside meeting place.
- If you cannot get out, stay in a room with the door closed and open the window for ventilation. Wave a bright-colored cloth or sheet out the window to signal to firefighters.

For more information on making a plan, go to pages 76–78.
For information on getting a kit for your family, go to pages 75–76.

FLOODS

Are You Ready for a Flood or a Flash Flood?

Here's what you can do to prepare for such emergencies.

Know What to Expect

Know your area's flood risk. If unsure, call your local American Red Cross chapter, emergency management office or planning and zoning department.
If it has been raining hard for several hours, or steadily raining for several days, be alert to the possibility of a flood.
Listen to local radio or TV stations or a NOAA Weather/All-Hazards Radio for flood information.

Reduce Potential Flood Damage By—

- Raising your furnace, water heater and electric panel if they are in areas of your home that may be flooded.
- Consult with a professional for further information on whether this and other damage-reduction measures can be taken.

FLOODING

Floods can take several hours to days to develop.
A FLOOD WATCH means a flood is possible in your area.
A FLOOD WARNING means flooding is already occurring or will occur soon in your area.

When a FLOOD WATCH is issued—

Move your furniture and valuables to higher floors of your home. Fill your car's gas tank in case an evacuation notice is issued.

When a FLOOD WARNING is issued—
Listen to local radio or TV stations or a NOAA Weather/All-Hazards Radio for information and advice. If told to evacuate, do so as soon as possible.

FLASH FLOODS
Flash floods can take only a few minutes to a few hours to develop.
A FLASH FLOOD WATCH means flash flooding is possible in your area.
A FLASH FLOOD WARNING means a flash flood is occurring or will occur very soon.

When a FLASH FLOOD WATCH is issued—
Be alert to signs of flash flooding and be ready to evacuate on a moment's notice.

When a FLASH FLOOD WARNING is issued—
Or if you think it has already started, evacuate immediately. You may have only seconds to escape. Act quickly! Move to higher ground away from rivers, streams, creeks and storm drains. Do not drive around barricades . . . they are there for your safety.

Make a Plan

- Check to see if you have insurance that covers flooding. If not, find out how to get flood insurance.
- Keep insurance policies, documents and other valuables in a safe deposit box.

Get a Kit
For information on getting a kit for your family, go to pages 75–76.

HURRICANES

Are You Ready for a Hurricane?

Here's what you can do to prepare for such an emergency.

Know What to Expect

Know your area's hurricane risk. If unsure, call your local American Red Cross chapter, National Weather Service office or emergency management office. Strong winds, storm surges and flooding, tornadoes and marine hazards are the greatest threats from hurricanes. Listen to local radio or TV stations or a NOAA Weather/All-Hazards Radio for severe weather information and leave if directed to do so by officials.

Reduce Potential Hurricane Damage By—

- Making a list of items to bring inside in the event of a storm.
- Removing any debris or loose items in your yard and keeping trees and shrubbery trimmed.
- Installing permanent hurricane shutters on windows and doors.
- Tying the roof to the mainframe of your home with metal straps.
- Preparing a "wind safe" room for use when you have not been asked to leave or evacuate.

If you live in an area prone to flooding, follow flood preparedness precautions. For more information on preparing for floods, go to pages 67–68. Hurricanes make take several days to weeks to develop. Take action now to be ready.

A HURRICANE WATCH means there is a threat of hurricane storm conditions within 36 hours.
A HURRICANE WARNING means that hurricane storm conditions are expected in 24 hours or less.
A hurricane storm local statement, issued by local National Weather Service offices, summarizes the watches, warnings, evacuation information and most immediate threats to an area.

When a Hurricane WATCH is issued—
Listen to local radio or TV stations or NOAA Weather/All-Hazards Radio for weather updates.
Review your disaster plan, keep informed and be ready to act if a warning is issued.

When a Hurricane WARNING is issued—
Complete your storm preparations and leave the threatened area if directed to do so by local officials.

Make a Plan

- Develop a hurricane evacuation plan.
- Discuss your plan to ensure that all family members know what to do if a hurricane threatens.
- Know where to go with your animals in case of evacuation. Evacuation shelters generally do not accept pets, except for service animals.

For more information on making a plan, go to pages 76–78.

Get a Kit
For information on getting a kit for your family, go to pages 75–76.

THUNDERSTORMS

Are You Ready for a Thunderstorm?

Here's what you can do to prepare for such an emergency.

Know What to Expect

Know your area's thunderstorm risk. If unsure, call your local American Red Cross chapter, National Weather Service office or emergency management office.
All thunderstorms are dangerous because they produce lightning.
Learn about your community's warning system for severe thunderstorms.
Strong thunderstorms can produce hail, down-bursts and straight-line winds, power outages and even tornadoes and floods.
For more information about preparing for tornadoes, go to pages 73–74.
For more information about preparing for floods, go to pages 67–68.

Reduce Potential Thunderstorm Damage By—

- Making a list of items and bringing them inside if a storm occurs.
- Removing any debris or loose items in your yard.
- Installing permanent shutters to cover windows.

Severe thunderstorms can develop quickly.
A SEVERE THUNDERSTORM WATCH means severe thunderstorms are possible in and near the watch area.
A SEVERE THUNDERSTORM WARNING means severe weather has been reported by spotters or indicated by radar.

If a Severe Thunderstorm WATCH is issued—

Listen to local radio or TV stations or a NOAA Weather/All-Hazards Radio for information and advice.

If a Severe Thunderstorm WARNING is issued—

- Draw the blinds and shades over windows and then stay away from them.
- Unplug appliances and avoid using them.
- Avoid using the telephone.
- Avoid taking a bath or shower, or running water for any purpose.
- Be prepared to go to the "safe place" in your home.
- Continue to listen to local radio or TV stations or a NOAA Weather/All-Hazards Radio for severe weather information.
- Listen for the sound of thunder.
- Even if there is no official warning, if you see the signs of a thunderstorm, take precautions.

Make a Plan

- Pick a safe place in the lowest level of your home and away from windows where family members can gather in case the weather becomes more threatening.

For more information on making a plan, go to pages 76–78.

Get a Kit

For information on getting a kit for your family, go to pages 75–76.

TORNADOES

Are You Ready for a Tornado?

Here's what you can do to prepare for such an emergency.

Know What to Expect

Know your area's tornado risk. If unsure, call your local American Red Cross chapter, National Weather Service office or emergency management office.
Tornadoes can strike quickly. Watch for tornado danger signs.
Learn about your community's warning system and pick a safe place to go ahead of time.
If you observe threatening weather conditions, listen to local radio or TV stations or a NOAA Weather/All-Hazards Radio for severe weather information.

Reduce Potential Tornado Damage By—

- Making a list of items and bringing them inside if a storm occurs.
- Keeping trees and shrubbery trimmed.
- Removing any debris or loose items in your yard.
- Installing permanent shutters to cover windows and strengthening garage doors.

Tornadoes can develop quickly and with little or no time for advance warning.
A TORNADO WATCH means that tornadoes are possible in and near the watch area.
A TORNADO WARNING means that a tornado has been sighted or indicated by weather radar.

When a Tornado WATCH is issued—
Listen to local radio and TV stations or NOAA Weather/All-Hazards Radio for weather updates. Review your disaster plan and be ready to act if a warning is issued or you suspect a tornado is approaching.

When a Tornado WARNING is issued—
Go immediately to your tornado-safe room. If there is no basement, go to a center hallway, bathroom or closet on the lowest floor. If you are in a vehicle, get out and move to shelter in a nearby sturdy building or lie flat in a low spot away from the vehicle.

Make a Plan

- Pick a safe place in the lowest level of your home and away from windows where family members could gather during a tornado.
- Conduct periodic tornado drills to ensure all family members know what to do if a tornado threatens.

For more information on making a plan, go to pages 76–78.

Get a Kit

For information on getting a kit for your family, go to pages 75–76.

BE RED CROSS READY

It is important that you be prepared for possible disasters and other emergencies. Natural or human–caused disasters can strike suddenly, at anytime and anywhere. There are three actions everyone can take that can help make a difference...

GET A KIT

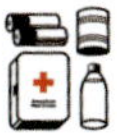

What you have on hand when a disaster happens can make a big difference. Have at least 3 days of supplies in an easy–to–carry evacuation kit, with additional supplies at home in case you cannot leave.

Remember to check your kit and replace the stock every 6 months.

An easy way to get your kit started is to contact your local American Red Cross or go online to www.redcross.org *to order your emergency preparedness kit today. If you purchase a kit or choose to build your own, check that it includes the following:*

Water: at least 1 gallon per person per day.
Food: non-perishable foods you enjoy that require no refrigeration, preparation or cooking and little or no water; may include high-protein items, including energy bars, ready-to-eat soup, peanut butter, etc.
Flashlight: include extra batteries or use an alternative energy option.
First aid kit: include a first aid reference guide.
Medications: include prescription and nonprescription medications, and copies of the prescriptions.
Radio: include extra batteries or use an alternative energy option.

Tools: wrench, manual can opener, screwdriver, hammer, pliers, knife, duct tape, plastic sheeting and garbage bags.
Clothing: a change of clothes for everyone, including sturdy shoes and work gloves.
Personal items: eyeglasses or contact lenses and solution; unique items for infants, seniors and people with disabilities.
Copies of important papers: including identification cards, insurance policies, birth certificates, passports, etc.
Comfort items: toys, books, etc.
Sanitary supplies: toilet paper, towelettes, feminine supplies, personal hygiene items, bleach, etc.
Money: cash and coins in case credit cards do not work.
Contact list: family phone numbers, e-mail addresses, meeting locations and out-of-area contact information.
Pet supplies: food, water, leash, litter box or plastic bags, tags, medications and vaccination information.
Map: including evacuation routes marked on it from your local area.

Store your disaster supplies in sturdy yet easy-to-carry containers. Keep a smaller version of the kit in your vehicle. If you become stranded or are not able to return home, having some items with you may make you more comfortable until help arrives.

MAKE A PLAN

Planning ahead is the first step to a more calm and more assured disaster response.

TALK. Discuss with your family the disasters that can happen where you live. Establish responsibilities for each member of your household and plan to work together as a team. Designate alternates in case someone is absent. If a family member is in the military, also plan for how you would respond if they are deployed and include the local military base resources that may be available.

PLAN. Choose two places to meet after a disaster:

- Right outside your home, in case of a sudden emergency, such as a fire.
- Outside your neighborhood, in case you cannot return home or are asked to evacuate your neighborhood.

LEARN. Each adult in your household should learn how and when to turn off utilities such as electricity, water and gas. Ask your local fire department to show you how to use a fire extinguisher.

TELL. Tell everyone in the household where emergency information and supplies are kept. Make copies for everyone to carry with them. Keep the information updated.

PRACTICE. Practice evacuating your home twice a year. Drive your planned evacuation route and plot alternate routes on a map in case main roads are impassable or gridlocked.

INCLUDE YOUR PETS. If you must evacuate, take your animals with you. If it is not safe for you, it is not safe for them.

SUPPORT YOUR COMMUNITY. Support your community plans by volunteering in the community and by giving blood.

More than one million Americans serve their communities. They come from all walks of life and backgrounds and are of all ages. Red Cross volunteers help people in emergencies; they teach first aid classes; organize blood drives; and translate so that non-English speakers can receive Red Cross services. They connect members of the armed forces stationed overseas with their families. Our vital community services are made possible by people like you. *Contact your local American Red Cross chapter and ask how you can help.*

Blood is needed in times of emergency, but the ongoing need is also great. Every two seconds someone needs a blood transfusion—cancer patients, accident victims, premature infants, people with chronic diseases. Your blood donation means so much to individuals who need it and you can help make a difference.

Giving blood does not take much time. During times of crisis and every day, each blood donation has the power to help save as many as three lives. But whole blood only has a shelf life of 42 days. That is why it is so important to be a regular and frequent donor. America needs to have an adequate blood supply available at all times to meet any of the challenges we might face. *Call 1-800-GIVE LIFE (1-800-448-3543) or visit* www.givelife.org, *and make an appointment to donate blood today.*

BE INFORMED

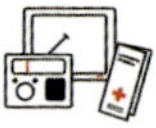

Knowing what may happen and how you can help may make all the difference when an emergency happens.

Learn what disasters or emergencies may occur where you live, work and play. These events can vary from only impacting you and your family — like a home fire or medical emergency — or your entire community — like an earthquake or flood. **Identify how local authorities will notify you** during a disaster and how you will get important information, including local radio, TV and NOAA weather radio.

Learn what you can do to prepare for these events by contacting your local American Red Cross chapter to ask about first aid, CPR and disaster training.

Learning simple first aid techniques can give you the skills and confidence to help anyone in your home, your neighborhood and at work. When a major disaster occurs, your community can change in an instant. Loved ones can be hurt and emergency response can be delayed. Make sure that at least one member of your household is trained in first aid and CPR and in how to use an AED. Disaster preparedness presentations will provide more specific information on how to prepare for disasters in your community. *Contact your local American Red Cross chapter for details.*

The three steps below can help you to react well in an emergency:

- **CHECK the scene** for safety and the victim for life-threatening conditions.
- **CALL 9-1-1** or your local emergency number and request professional assistance.
- **CARE for the victim** if you can reach the person safely.

Share what you have learned with your family, household and neighbors and encourage them to be informed too.

FIRST AID KIT CONTENTS

ACFAS MINIMUM RECOMMENDED FAMILY KIT CONTENTS—*Additional items may be added to personalize or customize this kit.*

Family First Aid Kit Content	Suggested Use
Absorbent Compress 5x9" dressing	Cover and protect open wounds
Adhesive Bandages (Assorted Sizes)	Cover and protect open wounds
Adhesive Tape (cloth) 1"	Secure bandages or splints
Antibiotic Ointment packets	Anti-infection (approx 1 g)
Antiseptic Wipe Packets	Wound cleaning/germ killing
Aspirin (Chewable) 81 mg	Symptoms of a heart attack**
Blanket (Space Blanket)	Maintain body temperature for shock
Breathing Barrier (w/ one-way valve)	Protection during rescue breathing/CPR
Instant Cold Compress	Control swelling
Gloves (lg), disposable, nonlatex	Prevent body fluid contact
Hydrocortisone Ointment Packets (approx 1 g)	External rash treatment
Scissors	Cut tape, cloth or bandages
Roller Bandage 3" (individually wrapped)	Secure wound dressing in place
Roller Bandage 4" (individually wrapped)	Secure wound dressing in place
Sterile Gauze Pad 3x3"	Control external bleeding
Sterile Gauze Pad 4x4"	Control external bleeding
Thermometer, Oral (Non-Mercury/Non-Glass)	Take temperature orally
Triangular Bandage	Sling or binder/splinting
Tweezers	Remove splinters or ticks
First Aid Instruction booklet	Self-explanatory

** 1. CALL 9-1-1 or the local emergency number. Never delay calling to administer aspirin.

2. If person is conscious, ask if he or she—
- Is allergic to aspirin.
- Has been advised by a physician not to take aspirin.
- Takes any blood thinners such as Coumadin™, warfarin or anti-platelet drugs.
- Has any stomach ulcer, disease or history of vomiting blood.

If the answer to any of the questions is "Yes," do not proceed with aspirin therapy.

3. If the answer to ALL four questions is "NO," the responder should offer 2 chewable (81 mg each) baby aspirins or 1 adult aspirin (325 mg). The above instructions do not constitute medical advice. Please seek medical advice prior to using any aspirin therapy.

FIRST AID This icon appears throughout this guide and denotes suggested items found in a First Aid Kit.